Finding the evidence: a gateway to the literature in child and adolescent mental health

SECOND EDITION

Gaskell is an imprint of the Royal College of Psychiatrists,
17 Belgrave Square, London SW1X 8PG, UK

British Library Cataloguing-in-Publication Data

A catalogue record for this book is available from the British Library.

ISBN 1–901242–68–4

The views presented in this book do not necessarily reflect those of the Royal College of Psychiatrists, and the publishers are not responsible for any error of omission or fact.

Gaskell is a registered trademark of the Royal College of Psychiatrists.

The Royal College of Psychiatrists is a registered charity (no. 228636).

Printed in the UK by Henry Ling Ltd, The Dorset Press, Dorchester.

Acknowledgements

The FOCUS Project is funded by a grant from the Gatsby Charitable Foundation and the Department of Health (Section 64 Grant award). The editors are grateful to the library staff of the Friends of the Children of Great Ormond Street Library, Sanjay Mistry and the Department of Epidemiology and Biostatistics at the Institute of Child Health for their support and assistance. We would also like to thank the contributors for both the first and second edition who provided references from their particular areas of expertise. Thanks also to Clare College, Cambridge, whose gates are pictured on the front cover.

Contents

Contributors

Dr Anthony Bailey (autism)
Clinical Scientist and Honorary Consultant in Child and Adolescent Psychiatry, Institute of Psychiatry, 16 De Crespigny Park, Denmark Hill, London SE5 8AF

Dr Derek Bolton (obsessive–compulsive disorder)
Department of Psychology, Institute of Psychiatry, De Crespigny Park, Denmark Hill, London SE5 8AF

Dr Domenico Di Ceglie (gender identity disorders)
Consultant Child and Adolescent Psychiatrist, Adolescent Department, Tavistock Clinic, 120 Belsize Lane, London NW3 5BA; Director, Gender Identity Development Unit, Portman Clinic; Honorary Senior Lecturer, Royal Free and University College Medical School, London

Dr David Coghill (psychopharmacology)
Senior Lecturer/Honorary Consultant, Ninewells Hospital, Department of Psychiatry, Dundee DD1 9SY

Dr Mary Eminson (somatoform disorders)
Consultant, NHS Child and Family Services, Royal Bolton Hospital, Farnworth, Bolton BL5 0JR

Dr Eric Fombonne (self-harm)
Reader in Epidemiological Child Psychiatry, MRC Child Psychiatry Unit, Institute of Psychiatry, 16 De Crespigny Park, Denmark Hill, London SE5 8AF

Professor Elena Garralda (chronic fatigue syndrome)
Professor in Child and Adolescent Psychiatry, Imperial College School of Medicine, St Mary's Campus, Norfolk Place, London W2 1PG

Dr Anne Gilchrist (Asperger's syndrome)
Consultant Adolescent Psychiatrist/Honorary Senior Lecturer, Royal Cornhill Hospital, Cornhill Road, Aberdeen AB25 2ZH

Dr Danya Glaser (emotional and physical abuse)
Consultant Child and Adolescent Psychiatrist, Department of Psychological Medicine, Great Ormond Street Hospital for Children, Great Ormond Street, London WC1N 3JH

Mr Anthony Harbour (legal issues)
Solicitor, Scott, Moncreiff, Harbour, Sinclair Solicitors, Signet House, 49–51 Farringdon Road, London EC1M 3JB

Professor Richard Harrington (depression)
Professor of Child and Adolescent Psychiatry, Royal Manchester Children's Hospital, Hospital Road, Charlestown Road, Pendlebury, Manchester M27 4HA

Mr Mike Heimann (group therapy)
Senior Clinical Nurse Specialist, Child and Adolescent Mental Health Services, Clare House, Blackshaw Road, London SW17 0QT

Professor Peter Hill   (attention-deficit hyperactivity disorder)
Consultant Child and Adolescent Psychiatrist, Department of Psychological
Medicine, Great Ormond Street Children's Hospital, Great Ormond Street, London
WC1N 3JH

Dr Peter Hindley   (child mental health and deafness)
Department of Child Psychiatry, Jenner Wing, St George's Hospital Medical
School, Cranmer Terrace, London SE17 0RE

Professor Chris Hollis   (schizophrenia)
Professor of Child and Adolescent Psychiatry, Developmental Psychiatry Section,
University Hospital, Nottingham NG7 2UH

Dr Ciaran Kelly   (elimination)
Consultant Child and Family Psychiatrist, Behaviour Resource Service,
315 Coxford Road, Lordswood, Southampton, Hampshire SO16 5LH

Dr Sebastian Kraemer   (consultation)
Consultant Child and Adolescent Psychiatrist, Tavistock Clinic and Whittington
Hospital, Child and Family Department, Tavistock Clinic, 120 Belsize Lane, London
NW3 5BA. sebastian@kraemer-zurne.freeserve.co.uk

Professor Bryan Lask   (eating disorders)
Reader, Eating Disorders Research Team, St George's Hospital Medical School,
Department of Psychiatry, Cranmer Terrace, Tooting, London SW17 0RE

Ms Cynthia Maynerd   (family therapy)
Head of Family Therapy, Cotswold House, Sutton Hospital, Cotswold Road, Surrey
SM2 5NF

Dr Julian Morrell   (conduct disorder)
Clinical Lecturer and Honorary Specialist Registrar, University Section of Child and
Adolescent Psychiatry, Park Hospital for Children, Old Road, Headington, Oxford
OX3 7LQ

Dr Martin Newman   (post-traumatic stress disorder)
Consultant Child Psychiatrist, William Harvey Clinic, 313–315 Cortis Road, Putney,
London SW15 6XG

Dr Sharon Pettle   (dying child)
Consultant Clinical Psychologist, Child and Family Consultation Centre,
1 Wolverton Gardens, London W6 7DQ

Dr Paul Ramchandani   (ethnicity in child and adolescent mental health)
Specialist Registrar, Section of Child and Adolescent Psychiatry, University of
Oxford Department of Psychiatry, Warneford Hospital, Headington, Oxford OX3 7JX

Dr Peter Reder   (parenting assessment)
Consultant Child Psychiatrist, Child and Family Consultation Centre, 1 Wolverton
Gardens, London W6 7DQ

Ms Jacqueline Robarts   (music therapy)
Nordoff Robbins Music Therapy Centre, 2 Lissenden Gardens, London NW5 1PP

Professor Mary Robertson   (Gilles de la Tourette syndrome)
Royal Free and University College London Medical School, Department of
Psychiatry and Behavioural Sciences, Wolfson Building, 48 Riding House Street,
London W1N 8AA; The National Hospital for Neurology and Neurosurgery, Queen
Square, London WC1N 8BG

Ms Margaret Rustin   (psychodynamic therapy)
Head of Child Psychotherapy, The Tavistock Clinic, 120 Belsize Lane, London
NW3 5BA

Dr Gill Salmon   (bullying)
Consultant in Child and Adolescent Psychiatry and Senior Lecturer in Child and
Adolescent Mental Health (University of Glamorgan), Trehafod Child and Family
Clinic, Waunarlwydd Road, Sketty, Swansea SA2 0GB

Dr Paramala Santosh   (mania and schizophrenia)
Lecturer in Child and Adolescent Psychiatry, Institute of Psychiatry, De Crespigny
Park, Denmark Hill, London SE5 8AF

**Ms Helen Shaw   (substance misuse and prevention, education and mental
health promotion)**
Policy Consultant in Health Education, Health Promotion and Adolescent Health,
362 Tinakori Road, Thornton, Wellington 6001, New Zealand.
helen.shaw@xtra.co.nz

Dr Howard Steele   (attachment)
Senior lecturer in Psychology, Director of the Attachment Research Unit,
Subdepartment of Clinical Health Psychology, University College London, 1–19
Torrington Place, London WC1E 7JD. h.steele@ucl.ac.uk

Dr Derek Steinberg   (consultation)
Consultant Psychiatrist, Adolescent Service and Young People's Unit, Ticehurst
House Hospital, Ticehurst, Nr Wadhurst, Sussex TN5 7HU

Dr Judith Trowell   (sexual abuse)
Consultant Psychiatrist, Child and Family Department, Tavistock Clinic, 120 Belsize
Lane, London NW3 5BA

Dr Garry Wannan   (mania)
Specialist Registrar, The Adolescent Service, 32 York Road, London SW11 3QJ

Professor Simon Wessely   (chronic fatigue syndrome)
Professor of Epidemiological and Liaison Psychiatry, Institute of Psychiatry,
Denmark Hill, London SE5 8AF

Mr Richard White   (legislation)
White and Sherwin Solicitors, Simpson House, 2–6 Cherry Orchard Road,
Croydon, Surrey CR0 6BA.

Dr Ian Wilkinson   (anxiety and phobia)
Consultant Clinical Psychologist, CAMHS Service, William Brown Centre, Manor
Way, Peterlee, Co. Durham SR85 5TW

Dr Ann York   (depression)
Consultant Child and Adolescent Psychiatrist, Child and Family Consultation
Centre, Richmond Royal Hospital, Kew Foot Road, Richmond, Surrey TW7 2TE

Introduction: the editors' goals and plans

There is an unprecedented demand for scientific evidence in child and adolescent mental health. Clinicians are under pressure to keep up to date and demonstrate that their decisions are based on the best available evidence. Families are hungry for information about their children's difficulties and what they can do to help or get help. Similarly, policy-makers and health service commissioners need a rational basis for prioritising service developments.

Electronic tools, such as the Internet, offer immediate access to a huge and rapidly expanding child and adolescent mental health literature. Without a critical guide there is a danger of being overwhelmed by the sheer volume of information.

Finding the Evidence is a unique type of publication, with three main aims: first, to identify the best available scientific evidence, second, to promote critical appraisal, and finally, to be scrupulously up to date. In essence, *Finding the Evidence* aims to promote evidence-based practice by providing the best available evidence where possible on the topics covered.

As in the first edition, the second edition of *Finding the Evidence* was compiled using two methods to select the evidence. First, electronic search strategies were applied to identify all relevant systematic reviews, meta-analyses and practice parameters or clinical guidelines. Second, experts were asked to choose (non-systematic) reviews, cutting edge and classic papers and books. The introductory sections are a new addition to the second edition.

As the term implies, systematic reviews weigh the evidence using systematic criteria to minimise error and bias. Meta-analyses merge and re-analyse the results of studies that are sufficiently similar and robust. Clinical guidelines should be systematically developed for use in specific clinical situations.

High-quality systematic reviews, meta-analyses and clinical guidelines are, scientifically, extremely valuable. Unfortunately, this type of systematic evidence is very limited in the child and adolescent mental health literature. For this reason, we have included all the systematic reviews, meta-analyses and clinical guidelines found (see comments below about critical appraisal and future editions).

Readers are invited to let us know about any systematic reviews, meta-analyses and clinical guidelines we have overlooked. (There is a form at the back of the book, or contact us at FOCUS.)

To explore the literature further, we have taken advice from researchers, academics and practitioners with a special interest in each field. This has been the basis on which we have selected reviews, where the evidence has been weighed on the basis of the author's personal opinion, rather than explicit systematic criteria. Cutting edge papers present important new theories and evidence, while classic papers are landmark publications of enduring interest. We also posed two critical questions to the experts, which we hope will be useful in highlighting pertinent issues in the field.

Not all topics fit neatly into this framework and we have been flexible where appropriate. For example, we have used very different headings for the section on consent to treatment. Scientific evidence is developing much more quickly and is far more advanced in some areas. Thus, while a paper on suicide published in 1996 is considered a classic, the scientific literature on music therapy is at a much earlier stage of development. We have been extremely fortunate in receiving advice from internationally renowned experts and in some areas advice from more than one expert. We are keen to extend the range of expert advice in the future.

No list can be exhaustive and *Finding the Evidence* points readers in the right direction. Part 1 provides guidance on finding evidence, while Part 2 presents the evidence on individual conditions, treatment approaches, emerging data-sets, and service development and legal issues.

All evidence needs to be critically examined, and Appendix ii provides a range of critical appraisal tools. Future electronic editions will include our own critical appraisals of the systematic reviews, meta-analyses and cutting edge papers cited in the book, using published criteria.

We are committed to keeping *Finding the Evidence* up to date, by continually renewing the searches, adding to the expert advice and acting on the suggestions of readers. The first edition of *Finding the Evidence* is already available at http://www. focusproject.org.uk (go to 'Completed work and available resources') and we hope to update this version with new material every six months. We are presently arranging for the cited articles to be critically appraised, and the electronic version will then contain the critical appraisals as they are completed. Ultimately, we hope that full text articles will be available using Internet links to the article's publishers.

We are very aware that there are gaps in the subject areas covered. We have tried in this edition of *Finding the Evidence* to include more subject areas than the first edition and will continue to include more subject areas in future editions. We would value readers' views on what to include.

Finding the Evidence will be of most value to clinicians, trainees and policy-makers. However, as more topic areas are covered, *Finding the Evidence* will become more relevant to all disciplines contributing to child and adolescent mental health care, as well as to carers and/or relatives.

We envisage *Finding the Evidence* as a 'living document', evolving to address the growing demand for knowledge and exploit the new opportunities provided by information technology.

Angela Scott, Mike Shaw & Carol Joughin

Angela Scott is currently the Information Officer for the FOCUS Project at the Royal College of Psychiatrists' Research Unit. She has an Honours degree in Applied Psychology and a background in psychometric testing.

Mike Shaw is a consultant child and adolescent psychiatrist at South West London and St George's Mental Health NHS Trust, where he runs the Stepping Stones in-patient unit for pre-adolescent children (Cotswold House, Sutton Hospital, Costwold Road, Surrey SM2 5NF). He is also an Honorary Senior Lecturer at St George's Hospital Medical School and Programme Director for the local Child and Adolescent Higher Specialist Training Scheme.

Carol Joughin leads the FOCUS Project. She has a background in both primary and secondary health care, having worked as a clinician, manager and researcher in a wide variety of health care settings.

Part 1
A guide to finding the evidence

Section 1: a description of terms

Evidence-based practice and the hierarchy of evidence

Evidence-based practice is often defined as the "conscientious, explicit and judicious use of the current best evidence in making decisions about the care of individual patients".[1] Evidence-based practice involves the use of skills whereby new evidence is located, examined and integrated into services and for the care of individual patients.[2]

The traditional hierarchy of evidence is as follows: several systematic reviews of randomised controlled trials (RCTs) or meta-analyses, systematic review of RCTs, RCTs, quasi-experimental trials, case-control and cohort studies, expert consensus opinion and finally individual opinion. It is important to recognise that the evidence that is searched for should not only depend on this hierarchy of evidence but also on the question that you are asking. It may well be the case that there are no systematic reviews in the area that you are searching for and other forms of evidence may be more appropriate.

Clinical Evidence

Clinical Evidence is a compendium of evidence on the effects of common clinical interventions, published every six months in book form and electronically by the BMJ Publishing Group. It summarises the best available evidence and highlights areas where there is little good evidence. Clinical Evidence provides a concise account of the current state of knowledge on a range of clinical conditions based on thorough searches of the literature. It is not a textbook of medicine or a book of guidelines.

Each issue of Clinical Evidence updates and expands its coverage. In each subject area in *Finding the Evidence*, we have indicated the chapter reference in Clinical Evidence if applicable, and in some cases whether it is going to be an area covered in future editions.

See http://www.evidence.org.

Systematic reviews

The term 'systematic review' implies that a review has been prepared using a systematic approach to minimise bias and random errors. Systematic reviews differ from other reviews in that they adhere to a documented, transparent structure. Rather than reflecting the views of the author or a selection of published literature, they should be

---

1   Sackett D, Rosenberg W, Gray J A M, *et al* (1996) Evidence based medicine: What it is and what it isn't. *British Medical Journal*, **312**, 71–72.
2   Ramchandani P, Joughin C & Zwi M (2001) Evidence-based child and adolescent mental health services – oxymoron or brave new dawn? *Child Psychology and Psychiatry Review*, **6**, 59–64.

comprehensive.[3] They aim to establish whether scientific findings are consistent and can be generalised across populations and whether the findings differ significantly by particular subsets. Meta-analyses are undertaken in some systematic reviews if the data are considered to be robust and the studies are sufficiently similar in design to allow for the findings to be merged and re-analysed as a single cohort. However, the reader should be aware that not all researchers will have taken a systematic approach to the development of their meta-analysis and this can lead to significant bias.

It is important to note that we have not checked the quality of the systematic reviews or meta-analyses for this edition of *Finding the Evidence*. We hope to have all of these papers critically appraised, which will help to identify systematic reviews and meta-analyses of poor quality. We have, however, provided tools in Appendix ii that will help you to appraise the quality of the research yourself.

For the purposes of this list, we have searched Medline, PsychINFO and the Cochrane Library for systematic reviews and meta-analyses using defined search strategies (see Appendix i). For this edition, we re-searched all Medline and PsychINFO from 1980 to 1999 using a high-precision, low-sensitivity search strategy, and a high-sensitivity, low-precision search strategy for the year 2000. The systematic reviews that have been found on the Cochrane database have been checked by Cochrane to meet the criteria of a high-quality systematic review. Articles containing systematic reviews that have been reviewed in the Database of Abstracts of Reviews of Effectiveness (DARE) are indicated in the references and have met the criteria for a systematic review. The review can be viewed in the Cochrane Database.

More about Cochrane

The Cochrane Collaboration is an international organisation that aims to help people make well-informed decisions about health care by preparing, maintaining and promoting the accessibility of systematic reviews of the effects of health care interventions. The Cochrane Collaboration produces the Cochrane Library, which is a collection of databases, published on-line as well as on disc and CD-ROM, which are updated on a quarterly basis. The Cochrane Library consists of the Cochrane Database of Systematic Reviews (CDSR), the DARE, the Cochrane Controlled Trials Register (CCTR) and the Cochrane Review Methodology Database.

- The CDSR is the main product of the Cochrane Collaboration. It brings together all the currently available Cochrane Reviews and also gives details of protocols for systematic reviews that have been registered with the Cochrane Collaboration. You can be certain that systematic reviews produced under the Cochrane Collaboration will have met the stringent criteria for systematic reviews. Where available, we have included protocols for systematic reviews under the individual conditions and treatment approaches.

- The DARE is a collection of abstracts of quality-assessed systematic reviews, other assessed reviews and bibliographic references. The DARE is produced by the NHS Centre for Reviews and Dissemination at the University of York.

- The CCTR includes references to clinical trials compiled by the Cochrane Review Groups. These trials have been judged as meeting certain quality standards.

See the Cochrane Collaboration at http://www.cochrane.org or the Cochrane Library at http://www.update-software.com/cochrane/cochrane-frame.html.

---

3   University of York NHS Centre for Reviews and Dissemination, 1996.

Collaborative Review Groups

Cochrane Collaborative Review Groups consist of individuals who share an interest in a particular area of health care. Their main purpose is to prepare and maintain systematic reviews of relevance to the group. The main collaborative review group of relevance to child and adolescent mental health is the Developmental, Psychosocial and Learning Problems Group. They plan to address a range of medical, social, educational and socio-legal problems that will cover: developmental and psycho-social problems of childhood and adolescence, including juvenile delinquency; learning problems (including, but not restricted to learning disabilities) and personality disorders and adult offending.

Where possible, sections in this resource give the contact name and details for the relevant Cochrane Collaborative Review Group.

Practice parameters

The practice parameters published in the *Journal of the American Academy of Child and Adolescent Psychiatry* are developed through peer review and provide the Academy's guidelines for the generally accepted level of practice, including guidelines for grade school-aged children, pre-school children and adolescents. See http://www.aacap.org.

Guidelines

These consist of a series of systematically developed statements to assist patients and practitioners when making decisions about appropriate health care in specified clinical circumstances. They should be based on information from systematic reviews and incorporate the views of clinicians and patients. However, not all clinical guidelines have been developed using a robust approach and readers should therefore use the critical appraisal tool in Appendix ii before using the information to inform their practice.

A list of databases of critically appraised guidelines is available at http://www.ihs.ox.ac.uk/libary/librarylinks.htm#guidelines.

Classic and cutting edge papers

Cutting edge papers present important new theories and evidence, while classic papers are landmark publications of enduring interest. We relied on the contributors for each section to select what they perceived to be the most relevant papers for these sections. Thus, in cases where there are new contributors for subject areas, the cutting edge and classic papers may vary in each edition.

Medline

Medline is compiled by the National Library of Medicine of the United States and indexes over 4000 journals published in over 70 countries. It lists about 300,000 articles per year and covers all areas of medicine, including nursing, psychiatry, psychology, biochemistry and health care management. It does not include books or conference abstracts (even if they are printed in journals indexed on Medline). Medline is available in three forms:

- ❍ a printed version: the Index Medicus;

- ❍ on-line: from 1996 to date – this can be accessed on the Internet by a number of servers; and

- ❍ CD-ROM: this may be accessed in libraries on between 10 and 18 CDs. Many trusts have also made it available through the local networks to offices and clinical areas.

See http://omni.ac.uk/medline.

PsychINFO (formally known as PsychLIT)

PsychINFO is a computerised CD-ROM database produced by a division of the American Psychological Association. PsychINFO covers the professional and academic field of psychology and related disciplines, including medicine, psychiatry, nursing, sociology, education, pharmacology, physiology and linguistics. The coverage is worldwide and includes references from 1887. PsychoINFO provides access to references and/or abstracts for international journal articles and book chapters. See http://www.apa.org/psycinfo.

EMBASE

EMBASE is a bibliographic database, produced by Excerpta Medica, a division of Elsevier Science Publishers B.V. It is a biomedical database that covers around 3500 journals from 110 countries from 1980 onwards. EMBASE's particular strengths are in the fields of drug research, pharmacology and toxicology. EMBASE also contains a thesaurus called EMTREE, which is a powerful tool for searching. EMBASE is updated monthly and is accessed via an OVID interface. See http://www.silverplatter.com/catalog/embx.htm.

Section 2: a guide to searching

The evidence listed in sections 5–8 provides a starting point of relevant research information for various topics. If you wish to search for more information we would suggest the following approach. Please remember that this is a very basic guide and is not a substitute for a training session with your local librarian!

○ **Step 1. Medline and PsychINFO search**
These are still the best databases to start with. However, for general therapy questions, the Cochrane Library now contains more controlled trials than Medline. For systematic reviews and meta-analyses, use the search strategy given in Appendix i. If you are doing a more extensive search remember to look in EMBASE. This will give you a wider choice of European journals.

○ **Step 2. Cochrane Library**
This is available on CD-ROM and will give you access to systematic reviews, protocols for systematic reviews in development, information from the DARE and primary studies from the CCTR.

○ **Step 3. Clinical practice guidelines**
For clinical practice guidelines, try the National Guideline Clearing House: http://www.guidelines.gov.index.asp. Also, check the Scottish Intercollegiate Guidelines Network: http://www.show.scot.nhs.uk/sign/index.html or for critically appraised guidelines visit http://www.ihs.ox.ac.uk/library/library links.htm#guidelines for a list of useful sites.

More about Medline

A number of different companies sell Medline and so slightly different commands are required depending on the supplier. Two of the most common suppliers are Ovid Technologies (OVID) and Silver Platter Information Ltd (WinSPIRS).

Ways of searching

You can search for articles in two ways:

1. By text word: This will give you any word that is listed on the database. It will include the title, abstract and authors' names or institute where the research was performed.

2. By MeSH heading. Medline and PsychINFO use a thesaurus to make searching more effective. A thesaurus is a controlled vocabulary that is used to index information from journals. It groups related concepts using a single preferred term. Medline and the Cochrane Library both use a thesaurus called MeSH. MeSH contains approximately 17,000 terms. Each term represents a single concept appearing in the literature. Using OVID, MeSH headings can be identified using a 'mapping' procedure. When using SilverPlatter, they can be identified by checking the thesaurus or using the

'suggest' option. Sometimes, you will not be able to find a MeSH term to match your subject. If this is the case, you will need to search using textwords. However, do remember that when searching on textwords the database will be searched for exactly the term that you have entered. You will, therefore, need to remember to consider all possible spellings and terms to describe your subject.

Exploding!

MeSH terms are arranged in hierarchical structures called trees. They start with a broad term and divide into branches of more specific terms.

TABLE 1.   EXAMPLE OF A MESH TREE

o   Eating disorders

     o   Anorexia nervosa

     o   Hyperphagia

          o   Bulimia

     o   Pica

Database indexers are instructed to use the most specific term(s) available when indexing papers. During the mapping process, you will first be offered the most general term and then the more specific term (if available). The tree structure allows you to explode your search. Exploding helps you obtain comprehensive coverage of your subject area. You can search for your MeSH term plus all its narrower terms at the same time.

Major headings

As many as 20 MeSH terms are assigned by indexers to any one article. Some headings are designated as major headings; these represent the main concepts of a paper. These major headings are prefaced by an asterisk (*) and help distinguish articles that discuss your subject in detail from those that discuss it briefly.

Boolean operators

Boolean operators can be used to combine keywords in your search strategy. AND allows you to link together different subjects; it focuses your search and allows you to retrieve fewer papers. For example, by searching for sexual abuse AND conduct disorder, you will only identify papers that address both issues together. OR allows you to broaden your search. If you search for sexual abuse OR conduct disorder, you will identify papers that address either sexual abuse or conduct disorder or both issues.

NOT should be used with care but could be used to identify papers that, for example, address hyperkinetic disorder but not conduct disorder (hyperkinetic disorder NOT conduct disorder).

Further refining your search

The abstract may be searched for areas of interest in the text, for example inserting random* will pick up 'randomised', 'randomized', 'randomisation' and 'randomization' if you are looking for an RCT.

Searching for terms in a particular field (e.g. author or title)

If you are trying to track down a paper and you know a few details you can search by using field suffixes such as:

.ab   Word in abstract

.au   Author

.pt   Publication type

.sh   Subject heading (MeSH)

.tw   Word in title or abstract

These are OVID suffixes, but the ones in SilverPlatter are very similar.

EXAMPLE

If you are looking for a paper on child sexual abuse and you know it was published in the *Journal of the American Academy of Child and Adolescent Psychiatry* simply enter:

1. Child sexual abuse.ti
   .ti shows that the term is in the title

2. Journal of the American Academy of Child and Adolescent Psychiatry.jn
   .jn shows that this is the journal you are looking for

3. Then combine the two instructions #1 AND #2

Sensitivity and specificity

Sensitivity is the likelihood of retrieving 'relevant' items; specificity is the likelihood of excluding 'irrelevant' items. To increase the sensitivity and so increase the records retrieved:

○ Broaden your question.

○ Try to use more search terms (look at the papers that you already have and see what they have used).

○ Use truncation (* or $) in textword searches.

- Add in and combine terms of related meaning using OR.
- Use the word NEAR to retrieve terms in the same sentence.
- Use the 'explode' feature.
- Select 'all subheadings' with MeSH terms.
- Extend the dates of publication.

To increase the specificity of your search and so reduce the papers retrieved:

- Narrow your question.
- Use more specific terms in a textword search.
- Use MeSH terms rather than a textword search.
- Use more specific MeSH terms.
- Add in terms using AND to represent other areas of your question.
- Limit to a particular language or publication type, e.g. RCT or meta-analysis.

QUICK TIP

The search strategy in Appendix i will allow you to pick up the maximum possible number of RCTs. This can be saved on disc and used again and again for different searches. We have also provided a search strategy for systematic reviews and meta-analyses.

Search terms and truncation

At the end of each section we have added suggested search terms and the number of primary research papers that you will be able to access if you search on the CCTR. Always remember to try alternative spellings for words such as 'behaviour'; using 'behavior' will usually generate many more hits. Other useful tips include using parentheses to link words together and using an asterisk to ensure that all words with the same beginning are included. For example, 'child*' will include child, child's and children.

References and suggested further reading

Greenhalgh T (1997) *How to Read a Paper: The Basics of Evidence-Based Medicine*. London: BMJ Publishing Group.

University of York NHS Centre for Reviews and Dissemination (1996) *Undertaking Systematic Reviews of Research on Effectiveness*. CRD Report No. 4. York: NHS Centre for Reviews and Dissemination.

Section 3: finding the evidence summary

1. Compose a clinical question. This should focus your search and ensure that it is appropriate.

Remember to define: (a) the population or type of patient (age, gender, diagnosis etc.); (b) the intervention or exposure; and (c) the outcome of interest.

EXAMPLE

In girls between the ages of 3 and 9 years with conduct disorder, do parent training programmes improve the child's attendance at school?

2. Identify relevant databases to search.

Consider Medline, Psychlit, the Cochrane Library and also sites such as the Health Technology Assessment site for key reports and the National Guideline Clearing House for clinical guidelines (see Step 3 in previous section).

3. Identify search terms for each component of the question. Always remember possible alternative spellings and terms.

Remember to use textwords and MeSH headings.

EXAMPLE

When searching for conduct disorder, also consider using: behavioural problem*, antisocial behaviour, antisocial behavior and behaviour disorder*.

4. Determine your Boolean operators, such as AND, OR and NOT.

These allow you to define the papers that you are interested in.

EXAMPLE

If you are looking for papers that discuss girls and not boys with hyperkinetic disorder you could put: child* AND girl* NOT boy* AND hyperkinetic disorder.

5. Adjust your search strategy to further limit the search if you have too many citations, or broaden it if you have too few.

Consider limiting to English language or a more specific term for the condition. See the section on sensitivity and specificity.

Part 2
The evidence

Section 4: directory

This section is organised by diagnostic categories and therapeutic approaches. The evidence is presented through systematic reviews, meta-analyses, clinical guidelines, practice parameters, reviews, reports and cutting edge and classic papers. Suggestions on where to find out more about specific topics are also included.

This directory lists diagnostic categories and therapeutic approaches by frequently used terms, in alphabetical order. These terms will direct the reader to the appropriate section.

ADD	see ATTENTION-DEFICIT HYPERACTIVITY DISORDER
ADHD	see ATTENTION-DEFICIT HYPERACTIVITY DISORDER
abnormal illness behaviour	see PAEDIATRIC LIAISON: somatoform disorder
abuse	see ABUSE: emotional and physical, and ABUSE: sexual
affective disorders	see EMOTIONAL DISORDERS: depression, and PSYCHOSIS: mania, and bipolar affective disorder
aggression	see CONDUCT DISORDERS AND JUVENILE DELINQUENCY
alcohol	see SUBSTANCE MISUSE
amphetamines	see ATTENTION-DEFICIT HYPERACTIVITY DISORDER
anorexia nervosa	see EATING DISORDERS
antidepressant drugs	see EMOTIONAL DISORDERS: depression
antisocial behaviour	see CONDUCT DISORDERS AND JUVENILE DELINQUENCY
anxiety	see EMOTIONAL DISORDERS: anxiety and phobia
Asperger's syndrome	see PERVASIVE DEVELOPMENT DISORDERS: Asperger's syndrome
assessment	see EMERGING DATA-SETS: assessment
attachment disorders	see EMERGING DATA-SETS: attachment disorders
attention-deficit hyperactivity disorder	see ATTENTION-DEFICIT HYPERACTIVITY DISORDER
autism	see PERVASIVE DEVELOPMENTAL DISORDERS: autism, and PAEDIATRIC LIAISON: dementia

17

behavioural problems	see CONDUCT DISORDERS AND JUVENILE DELINQUENCY
bipolar affective disorder	see PSYCHOSIS: mania and bipolar affective disorder
body image	see EATING DISORDERS
brain disorders	see PAEDIATRIC LIAISON: dementia
bulimia nervosa	see EATING DISORDERS
CAMHS	see SERVICE DEVELOPMENT AND LEGAL ISSUES: organisation of CAMHS
challenging behaviour	see CONDUCT DISORDERS AND JUVENILE DELINQUENCY
child mental health services	see SERVICE DEVELOPMENT AND LEGAL ISSUES: organisation of CAMHS
child protection	see SERVICE DEVELOPMENT AND LEGAL ISSUES: parenting assessment; legislation
Children Act 1989	see SERVICE DEVELOPMENT AND LEGAL ISSUES: legislation; consent and competence
chronic fatigue syndrome	see PAEDIATRIC LIAISON: chronic fatigue syndrome
competence	see SERVICE DEVELOPMENT AND LEGAL ISSUES: consent and competence
compulsions	see EMOTIONAL DISORDERS: obsessive–compulsive disorder
conduct disorder	see CONDUCT DISORDERS AND JUVENILE DELINQUENCY
consent to treatment	see SERVICE DEVELOPMENT AND LEGAL ISSUES: consent and competence
constipation	see ELIMINATION
consultation	see SERVICE DEVELOPMENT AND LEGAL ISSUES: consultation
conversion disorder	see PAEDIATRIC LIAISON: somatoform disorder
court reports	see SERVICE DEVELOPMENT AND LEGAL ISSUES: legislation; parenting assessment
crime	see CONDUCT DISORDERS AND JUVENILE DELINQUENCY
deaf children	see EMERGING DATA-SETS: mental health and deafness
death	see PAEDIATRIC LIAISON: dying child
deliberate self-harm	see DELIBERATE SELF-HARM
delinquency	see CONDUCT DISORDERS AND JUVENILE DELINQUENCY

dementia	see PAEDIATRIC LIAISON: dementia
depression	see EMOTIONAL DISORDERS: depression
depressive feelings	see EMOTIONAL DISORDERS: depression
diagnosis	see EMERGING DATA-SETS: assessment
dieting	see EATING DISORDERS
disintegrative psychosis	see PAEDIATRIC LIAISON: disintegrative disorder
disruptive behaviour	see CONDUCT DISORDERS AND JUVENILE DELINQUENCY
drug abuse	see SUBSTANCE MISUSE
dying child	see PAEDIATRIC LIAISON: dying child
ECT	see EMERGING DATA-SETS: electroconvulsive therapy
eating disorders	see EATING DISORDERS
electroconvulsive therapy	see EMERGING DATA-SETS: electroconvulsive therapy
emotional abuse	see ABUSE: emotional and physical
emotional disorders	see EMOTIONAL DISORDERS
encephalitis	see PAEDIATRIC LIAISON: dementia
encopresis	see ELIMINATION
enuresis	see ELIMINATION
ethnic minorities	see EMERGING DATA-SETS: the mental health of children and adolescents from ethnic minorities
family therapy	see TREATMENT APPROACHES: family therapy
fatigue	see PAEDIATRIC LIAISON: chronic fatigue syndrome
fear	see EMOTIONAL DISORDERS: anxiety and phobia
gender identity disorders	see GENDER IDENTITY DISORDERS
Gilles de la Tourette syndrome	see TIC DISORDERS: tics and Gilles de la Tourette syndrome
glue-sniffing	see SUBSTANCE MISUSE
group therapy	see TREATMENT APPROACHES: group therapy
health services	see SERVICE DEVELOPMENT AND LEGAL ISSUES: organisation of CAMHS
heroin	see SUBSTANCE MISUSE
hyperactivity	see ATTENTION-DEFICIT HYPERACTIVITY DISORDER
hyperkinetic disorder	see ATTENTION-DEFICIT HYPERACTIVITY DISORDER

hypochondriasis	see PAEDIATRIC LIAISON: somatoform disorder
hypomania	see PSYCHOSIS: mania and bipolar affective disorder
infantile psychosis	see PERVASIVE DEVELOPMENT DISORDERS: autism
legislation	see SERVICE DEVELOPMENT AND LEGAL ISSUES: legislation; consent and competence
ME	see PAEDIATRIC LIAISON: chronic fatigue syndrome
mania	see PSYCHOSIS: mania and bipolar affective disorder
mental health services	see SERVICE DEVELOPMENT AND LEGAL ISSUES: organisation of CAMHS
mood disorders	see EMOTIONAL DISORDERS: anxiety and phobia, and EMOTIONAL DISORDERS: depression
music therapy	see TREATMENT APPROACHES: music therapy
myalgic encephalomyelitis	see PAEDIATRIC LIAISON: chronic fatigue syndrome
neglect	see ABUSE: emotional and physical
non-accidental injury	see ABUSE: emotional and physical
OCD	see EMOTIONAL DISORDERS: obsessive–compulsive disorder
ODD	see CONDUCT DISORDERS AND JUVENILE DELINQUENCY
obesity	see EATING DISORDERS
obsessional disorders	see EMOTIONAL DISORDERS: obsessive–compulsive disorder
oppositional defiant disorder	see CONDUCT DISORDERS AND JUVENILE DELINQUENCY
organisation of health services	see SERVICE DEVELOPMENT AND LEGAL ISSUES: organisation of CAMHS
overweightness	see EATING DISORDERS
PTSD	see POST-TRAUMATIC STRESS DISORDER
panic	see EMOTIONAL DISORDERS
parasuicide	see DELIBERATE SELF-HARM
parenting	see SERVICE DEVELOPMENT AND LEGAL ISSUES: parenting assessment
pervasive developmental disorder	see PERVASIVE DEVELOPMENT DISORDERS: autism, and PERVASIVE DEVELOPMENT DISORDERS: Asperger's syndrome
phobias	see EMOTIONAL DISORDERS: anxiety and phobia

physical abuse	see ABUSE: emotional and physical
post-traumatic stress disorder	see POST-TRAUMATIC STRESS DISORDER
prevention	see SERVICE DEVELOPMENT AND LEGAL ISSUES: prevention and mental health promotion
psychoanalysis	see TREATMENT APPROACHES
psychoses	see PSYCHOSIS: schizophrenia, and PSYCHOSIS: mania
psychotherapy	see TREATMENT APPROACHES: psychotherapy
psychopharmacology	see TREATMENT APPROACHES: psychopharmacology
refusal of treatment	see SERVICE DEVELOPMENT AND LEGAL ISSUES: consent and competence
Rett's syndrome	see PAEDIATRIC LIAISON: dementia
rituals	see EMOTIONAL DISORDERS: obsessive–compulsive disorder
SSRIs	see EMOTIONAL DISORDERS: depression
schizophrenia	see PSYCHOSIS: schizophrenia
selective serotonin reuptake inhibitors	see EMOTIONAL DISORDERS: depression
self-harm	see DELIBERATE SELF-HARM
services	see SERVICE DEVELOPMENT AND LEGAL ISSUES: organisation of CAMHS
sexual abuse	see ABUSE: sexual
soiling	see ELIMINATION
solvent abuse	see SUBSTANCE MISUSE
somatoform disorders	see PAEDIATRIC LIAISON: somatoform disorders
stimulant medication	see ATTENTION-DEFICIT HYPERACTIVITY DISORDER
stress	see POST-TRAUMATIC STRESS DISORDER
subacute sclerosing panencephalitis	see PAEDIATRIC LIAISON: subacute sclerosing panencephalitis
substance abuse	see SUBSTANCE MISUSE
suicide	see DELIBERATE SELF-HARM
tics	see TIC DISORDERS: tics and Gilles de la Tourette syndrome
Tourette syndrome	see TIC DISORDERS: tics and Gilles de la Tourette syndrome
tricyclic antidepressants	see EMOTIONAL DISORDERS: depression

21

Section 5: individual conditions

ABUSE: emotional and physical

INTRODUCTION

Physical abuse can be defined as any form of physical injury that is inflicted on a child knowingly, or that was not prevented by the guardian of a child.[4]

Emotional abuse is the persistent emotional ill treatment of a child that causes severe persistent adverse effects on the child's emotional development. Emotional abuse can include conveying to a child that they are unloved, worthless or inadequate, and can involve developmentally inappropriate expectations of the child. Emotional abuse can cause a child to frequently feel frightened or feel that they are in danger. Some degree of emotional abuse is involved in all types of ill treatment of a child, but it can also occur on its own.[5]

Eighteen per cent of registrations on the Child Protection Register are for emotional abuse and 29% for physical injury.[6] Emotional abuse and neglect frequently coexist with physical abuse or neglect, although emotional abuse and neglect are also found independently of other forms of child abuse and neglect. The number of unreported instances of abuse may be greater than reported to the Child Protection Registers. In a recent national study by the National Society for the Prevention of Cruelty to Children (NSPCC), it was estimated that 6% of young people surveyed were emotionally maltreated, and 7% suffered serious physical abuse.[7]

DIAGNOSIS AND AETIOLOGY

An essential criterion for the diagnosis of physical abuse is that there would have to be certainty, or at the very least, reasonable suspicion, that the injury was committed knowingly. Symptoms of physical abuse can include cuts, bruises, burns, fractures and various forms of poisoning.[8]

Children subjected to emotional abuse and neglect may display emotional, behavioural, cognitive, social and physical difficulties.[9] However, emotional abuse and neglect cannot be inferred from the child's difficulties that are not specific to the abuse. Nonetheless, the various pervasive maltreating parental interactions with the child are observable.

---

4   Phillips C (1993) **Child abuse and disorders of parenting**. In *Seminars in Child and Adolescent Psychiatry* (eds D Black & D Cottrell), pp. 218–232. London: Gaskell.

5   Department of Health (1999) *Working to Safeguard Children*. London: The Stationery Office.

6   Government Statistical Service (2001) *Children and Young People on Child Protection Registers*. London: Department of Health.

7   NSPCC (2000) *Child Maltreatment in the United Kingdom: A Study of the Prevalence of Child Abuse and Neglect*. London: NSPCC.

8   Skuse D & Bentovim A (1994) **Physical and emotional maltreatment**. In *Child and Adolescent Psychiatry: Modern Approaches* (eds M Rutter, E Taylor & L Hersov). 3rd edn. Oxford: Blackwell Scientific Publications.

9   Glaser D & Prior C (1999) Is the term child protection applicable to emotional abuse? *Child Abuse Review*, **6**, 315–329.

by Dr Dania Glaser

What developments have there been in the management of emotional and physical abuse?

There have not been any major developments in the management of emotional abuse and neglect other than those outlined in the Glaser & Prior (1997) paper about earlier recognition, especially in association with domestic violence, parental mental illness and parental drug and alcohol abuse.

With regard to physical abuse, there has been an increase in the understanding of the very harmmful effects of shaking babies.

What are the key messages from new research that are not being widely used?

There is delayed and under-recognition of emotional abuse and neglect.

REFERENCES

● SYSTEMATIC REVIEWS AND META-ANALYSES ●

Kaplan S J, Pelcovitz D & Labruna V (1999) **Child and adolescent abuse and neglect research: a review of the past 10 years. Part I: Physical and emotional abuse and neglect**. *Journal of the American Academy of Child and Adolescent Psychiatry*, **38**, 1214–1222.

Stevenson J (1999) **The treatment of the long-term sequelae of child abuse**. *Journal of Child Psychology and Psychiatry and Allied Disciplines*, **40**, 89–111.

● PRACTICE PARAMETERS ●

American Academy of Child and Adolescent Psychiatry (1997) **Practice parameters for the forensic evaluation of children and adolescents who may have been physically or sexually abused**. *Journal of the American Academy of Child and Adolescent Psychiatry*, **36** (suppl.), 37–56.

● REVIEWS ●

Cicchetti D & Nurcombe B (eds) (1991) **Special edition devoted to defining psychological maltreatment**. *Development and Psychopathology*, **3**, 1–124.

Cohn A D & Davro D (1987) **Is treatment too late: what ten years of evaluative research tells us**. *Child Abuse and Neglect*, **11**, 433–442.

Glaser D & Prior V (1997) **Is the term 'child protection' applicable to emotional abuse?** *Child Abuse Review*, **6**, 315–329.

Hart S, Binggeli N & Brassard M (1998) **Evidence for the effects for psychological maltreatment**. *Journal of Emotional Abuse*, **1**, 27–58.

Macmillan H L, MacMillan J H, Offord D R, *et al* (1994) **Primary prevention of child physical abuse and neglect: a critical review: I**. *Journal of Child Psychology and Psychiatry*, **34**, 835–836.

● CLASSIC PAPERS ●

Skuse D H (1984) **Extreme deprivation in early childhood: diverse outcomes for three siblings from an extraordinary family**. *Journal of Child Psychology and Psychiatry*, **25**, 523–541.

—— (1984) **Extreme deprivation in early childhood: theoretical issues and a comparative review**. *Journal of Child Psychology and Psychiatry*, **25**, 543–572.

● CUTTING EDGE PAPERS ●

Claussen A H & Crittenden P M (1991) **Physical and psychological maltreatment: relations among types of maltreatment**. *Child Abuse and Neglect*, **15**, 5–18.

Gibbons J, Gallagher B, Bell C, *et al* (1995) *Development after Physical Abuse in Early Childhood: a Follow-up Study of Children on Protection Registers*. Social Work Development Unit, University of East Anglia. Studies in Child Protection. London: HMSO.

● BOOKS ●

Briere J, Berliner L, Bulkley J A, *et al* (1996) *The ASPAC Handbook on Child Maltreatment*. Thousand Oaks, CA: Sage Publications.

Garabino J, Guttmann E & Seeley J (1986) *The Psychologically Battered Child*. San Francisco: Jossey-Bass.

Glaser D (1995) **Emotionally abusive experiences**. In **Assessment of Parenting: Psychiatric and Psychological Contributions** (eds P Reder & C Lucey), pp. 73–86. London: Routledge.

● USEFUL WEBSITES ●

Childline http://www.childline.org.uk

Kidscape http://www.kidscape.org.uk

National Children's Bureau http://www.ncb.org.uk

National Clearing House on Child Abuse and Neglect Information http://calib.com/nccanch

National Society for the Protection of Cruelty to Children http://www.nspcc.org.uk

● ON-LINE JOURNALS ●

Child Abuse and Neglect http://elsevier/nl//locate/chiabuneg

Cochrane Controlled Trials Register
29 hits (keywords: child* AND physical abuse)

Cochrane Developmental, Psychosocial and Learning Problems Group
Contact: Dr Jane Dennis, Bristol, UK. J.Dennis@bristol.ac.uk

ABUSE: sexual

INTRODUCTION

Sexual abuse can be defined as any sexual contact between an adult and a child who is sexually immature (i.e. incapable of consenting because of age or power differentials in the relationship) for the sexual gratification of the adult. Sexual contact can be made by the use of force, threat or deceit to gain the child's participation.[10]

Sexual abuse occurs at all ages but is more common between the ages of 8 and 12 years, although there is some evidence that the onset of sexual abuse in boys may occur earlier.[11]

The widely differing definitions of sexual abuse and different methods of data collection have made it difficult to calculate the prevalence of sexual abuse. Recently, in a national study by the NSPCC, it was found that in England up until March 2000, 30,300 children were on the protection registers. Of these, 5,600 were registered for sexual abuse. From the study, it was found that 1% of young people reported sexual abuse by a parent or carer and 6% by another relative.[12]

DIAGNOSIS AND AETIOLOGY

A diagnosis of sexual abuse can be made for any sexual contact between an adult and a sexually immature child for sexual gratification.

The behaviours that are associated with sexual abuse depend on the age of the child. For example, sexualised play and behaviour is found in children under six years old, anxiety-related symptoms and sexual preoccupation in 7–12-year-olds, and acting out, deliberate self-harm, anorexia nervosa, drug and alcohol misuse, and prostitution in teenagers.[13]

CRITICAL QUESTIONS

by Dr Judith Trowell

What developments have there been in the management of sexual abuse?

- The new guidance on interviewing children is out as a consultation paper entitled *Achieving Best Evidence in Criminal Proceedings. Guidance for Vulnerable or Intimidated Victims including Children*. This will hopefully improve practice and the court process.

- The new Human Rights Act has been implemented.

- The assessment framework for children in need.

---

10 Finkelhor & Korbin (1998) cited in Smith M & Bentovim A (1994) Sexual abuse. In *Child and Adolescent Psychiatry: Modern Approaches* (eds M Rutter, E Taylor & L Hersov). 3rd edn. Oxford: Blackwell Scientific Publications.

11 Bentovim A *et al* (1987); Research Team (1990); Monck *et al* (1993) cited in Smith M & Bentovim A (1994) Sexual abuse. In *Child and Adolescent Psychiatry: Modern Approaches* (eds M Rutter, E Taylor & L Hersov). 3rd edn. Oxford: Blackwell Scientific Publications.

12 NSPCC (2000) *Child Maltreatment in the United Kingdom: A Study of the Prevalence of Child Abuse and Neglect*. London: NSPCC.

13 Phillips C (1993) Child abuse and disorders of parenting. In *Seminars in Child and Adolescent Psychiatry* (eds D Black & D Cottrell), pp. 218–232. London: Gaskell.

What are the key messages from new research that are not being widely used?

○ Research by Tebbutt from W2[14] (Doctes team) shows that sexually abused children do not spontaneously recover from depression/anxiety over time. They need treatment.

○ Lanktree and Briere[15] show how patient-led treatment packages can be evaluated and lead to improvement.

REFERENCES

● SYSTEMATIC REVIEWS AND META-ANALYSES ●

Davis M K & Gidycz C A (2000) **Child sexual abuse prevention programs: a meta-analysis**. *Journal of Clinical Child Psychology*, **29**, 257–265.

De-Jong T I & Gorey K M (1996) **Short-term versus long-term group work with female survivors of childhood sexual abuse: a brief meta-analytic review**. *Social Work with Groups*, **19**, 19–27.

Dhaliwal G K, Gauzas L, Antonowicz D H, *et al* (1996) **Adult male survivors of childhood sexual abuse: Prevalence, sexual abuse characteristics, and long-term effects**. *Clinical Psychology Review*, **16**, 619–639.

Finkelhor D & Berliner L (1995) **Research on the treatment of sexually abused children: a review and recommendations**. *Journal of the American Academy of Child and Adolescent Psychiatry*, **34**, 1408–1423. (Reviewed on DARE.)

Fossati A, Madeddu F & Maffei C (1999) **Borderline personality disorder and childhood sexual abuse: a meta-analytic study**. *Journal of Personality Disorders*, **13**, 268–280.

Jones D & Ramchandani P (1999) ***Child Sexual Abuse***. Oxford: Radcliffe Medical Press.

Jumper S A (1995) **A meta-analysis of the relationship of child sexual abuse to adult psychological adjustment**. *Child Abuse Neglect*, **19**, 715–728.

Macdonald G, Ramchandani P, Higgins J, *et al* (2000) **Cognitive–behavioural interventions for sexually abused children**. Protocol for Cochrane Review. In *The Cochrane Library*, Issue 4. Oxford: Update Software.

Neumann D A, Houskamp B M, Pollock V E, *et al* (1996) **The long-term sequelae of childhood sexual abuse in women: a meta-analytic review of child maltreatment**. *Child Maltreatment: Journal of the American Professional Society on the Abuse of Children*, **1**, 6–16.

Reeker J, Ensing D & Elliott R (1997) **A meta-analytic investigation of group treatment outcomes for sexually abused children**. *Child Abuse and Neglect*, **21**, 669–680. (Reviewed on DARE.)

---

14 Tebbutt J, Swanston H, Oates R K, *et al* (1997) **Five years after child sexual abuse: persisting dysfunction and problems of prediction**. *Journal of the American Academy of Child and Adolescent Psychiatry*, **36**, 330–339.

15 Lanktree C B & Briere J (1995) **Outcome of therapy of sexually abused children: a repeated measures study**. *Child Abuse and Neglect*, **19**, 1145–1155.

Rind B & Tromovitch P (1997) **A meta-analytic review of findings from national samples on psychological correlates of child sexual abuse**. *Journal of Sex Research*, **34**, 237–255.

—, — & Bauserman R (1998) **A meta-analytic examination of assumed properties of child sexual abuse using college samples**. *Psychological Bulletin*, **124**, 22–53.

Rispens J, Aleman A & Goudena P P (1997) **Prevention of child sexual abuse victimization: a meta-analysis of school programs**. *Child Abuse and Neglect*, **21**, 975–987. (Reviewed on DARE.)

Tourigny M (1997) **Efficacite des interventions pour enfants abuses sexuellement: une recension des ecrits. (Treatment outcome for sexually abused children: A review of studies)**. *Revue Canadienne de Psycho Education*, **26**, 39–69. (Reviewed on DARE.)

West M (1998) **Meta-analysis of studies assessing the efficacy of projective techniques in discriminating child sexual abuse**. *Child Abuse and Neglect*, **22**, 1151–1166.

Wonderlich S A, Brewerton T D, Jocic J, *et al* (1997) **Relationship of childhood sexual abuse and eating disorders**. *Journal of the American Academy of Child and Adolescent Psychiatry*, **36**, 1107–1115.

● PRACTICE PARAMETERS ●

American Academy of Child and Adolescent Psychiatry (1997) **Practice parameters for the forensic evaluation of children and adolescents who may have been physically or sexually abused**. *Journal of the American Academy of Child and Adolescent Psychiatry*, **36** (suppl.), 37S–56S.

● REVIEWS ●

Alvarez A (1989) ***Child Sexual Abuse: the Need to Remember and the Need to Forget. The Consequences of Child Sexual Abuse***. Occasional papers No. 3. London: Association of Child Psychology and Psychiatry.

Beitchman J H, Zucker K J, Hood, J E, *et al* (1991) **A review of short term effects of child sexual abuse**. *Child Abuse and Neglect*, **15**, 537–556.

—, —, —, *et al* (1992) **A review of the long term effects of child sexual abuse**. *Child Abuse and Neglect*, **16**, 101–118.

Kendall-Tackett K A, William L M & Finkelhor D (1993) **Impact of sexual abuse on children: a review and synthesis of recent empirical studies**. *Psychological Bulletin*, **113**, 164–180.

Sinason V (1988) **Smiling, swallowing, sickening and stupefying. The effect of abuse on the child**. *Psychoanalytic Psychotherapy*, **3**, 97–111.

Stevenson J (1999) **The treatment of the long term sequalae of child abuse**. *Journal of Child Psychology and Psychiatry*, **40**, 89–111.

Trowell J (1997) **Child sexual abuse**. In ***Rooted Sorrows*** (ed. Hon. Justice Wall), pp. 20–23. Bristol: Family Law.

● CLASSIC PAPERS ●

Finkelhor D & Browne A (1985) **The traumatic impact of child sexual abuse: a conceptualisation**. *American Journal of Orthopsychiatry*, **55**, 530–541.

Fredrick W N, Grambsch P, Broughton D, *et al* (1991) **Normal sexual behaviour in children**. *Journal of Paediatrics*, **88**, 456–464.

McLeer S V, Deblinger E, Atkins M S, *et al* (1988) **Post traumatic stress disorder in sexually abused children**. *Journal of the American Academy of Child and Adolescent Psychiatry*, **27**, 650–654.

Summit R (1983) **The child sexual abuse accommodation syndrome**. *Child Abuse and Neglect*, **7**, 177–193.

● CUTTING EDGE PAPERS ●

Lanktree C & Briere J (1995) **Outcome for therapy of sexually abused children: a repeated measure study**. *Child Abuse and Neglect*, **19**, 329–334.

Skuse D, Bentovim A, Hodges J, *et al* (1998) **Risk factors for development of sexually abusive behaviour in sexually victimised adolescent boys**. *British Medical Journal*, **317**, 175–179.

Tebbutt J, Swanston H, Oates R K, *et al* (1997) **Five years after child sexual abuse, persisting dysfunction and problems of prediction**. *Journal of the American Academy of Child and Adolescent Psychiatry*, **36**, 330–339.

● REPORTS ●

Royal College of Psychiatrists (1993) *Child Psychiatry and Child Sexual Abuse*. CR24. London: Royal College of Psychiatrists.

Sharland E, Seal H, Croucher M, *et al* (1996) *Professional Intervention in Child Sexual Abuse*. London: HMSO.

● BOOKS ●

Bentovim A, Elton A, Hildebrand J, *et al* (1988) *Child Sexual Abuse in the Family*. London: Wright Butterworth Press.

Furniss T (1991) *Multi-Professional Handbook of Child Sexual Abuse*. London: Routledge.

Glaser D & Frosh S (1993) *Child Sexual Abuse*. 2nd edn. London: Macmillan.

Kemple R & Kemple H (1984) *The Common Secret Sexual Abuse of Children and Adolescents*. San Francisco: Freeman Press.

Segroi S (1982) *Handbook of Clinical Interventions in Child Sexual Abuse*. Lexington, MA : Lexington Books.

● USEFUL WEBSITES ●

Childline http://www.childline.org.uk

Kidscape http://www.kidscape.org.uk

National Children's Bureau http://www.ncb.org.uk

National Clearing House on Child Abuse and Neglect Information http://calib.com/nccanch

National Data Archive on Child Abuse and Neglect (NDACAN) http://www.ndacan.cornell.edu

National Society for the Protection of Cruelty to Children http://www.nspcc.org.uk

● ON-LINE JOURNALS ●

Child Abuse and Neglect http://elsevier/nl/locate/chiabuneg

Journal of Child Sexual Abuse http://bubl.ac.uk/journals/soc/jcsa

---

Cochrane Controlled Trials Register
86 hits (keywords: child* AND abuse* AND sex*)

Cochrane Developmental, Psychosocial and Learning Problems Group
Contact: Dr Jane Dennis, Bristol, UK. J.Dennis@bristol.ac.uk

INTRODUCTION

Attention-deficit hyperactivity disorder (ADHD) is a persistent pattern of inattention, hyperactivity and/or impulsivity that is more pronounced and extreme than is typically observed in individuals at a similar stage of development.[16]

ADHD is a broader concept than hyperkinetic disorder since it can include extreme overactivity/impulsivity alone or inattentiveness alone. But where ADHD (combined type) incorporating overactivity, impulsivity and inattentiveness is considered, there is little difference from hyperkinetic disorder.

ADHD occurs in between 3% and 5%[17] of the population and hyperkinetic disorder in approximately 1% of the population. Boys appear to be three times more likely to suffer from ADHD than girls.[18]

DIAGNOSIS AND AETIOLOGY

The onset of ADHD is by definition before the age of seven years, but the onset of ADHD usually occurs before the age of five.

According to the DSM–IV–TR for the diagnosis of ADHD to be made the symptoms must:

○ be present for at least six months and present in more than one situation;

○ be evident since an early age;

○ impair the child's functions; and

○ not be better explained by another disorder.

The ICD–10 diagnosis differs from that in the DSM–IV–TR in that the term 'hyperkinetic disorder' is used. The diagnostic criteria are more restrictive and stringent than those in the DSM–IV–TR.

Other conditions frequently co-exist with ADHD, such as oppositional defiant disorder, conduct disorder, anxiety disorder and depressive disorders.[19]

The aetiology of ADHD is uncertain. There is only limited evidence of a genetic component.[20]

---

16   American Psychiatric Association (2000) *Diagnostic and Statistical Manual of Mental Disorders*. 4th edn (DSM–IV–TR). Washington DC: APA.

17   Phillips C (1993) **Child abuse and disorders of parenting**. In *Seminars in Child and Adolescent Psychiatry* (eds D Black & D Cottrell), pp. 218–232. London: Gaskell.

18   Green M, Wong M, Atkins D, *et al* (1999) **Diagnosis of Attention Deficit/Hyperactivity Disorder**. Council on Scientific Affairs, American Medical Association. Technical Review No. 3. (prepared by Technical Resources International, Inc. under contract no 290-94-2024). AHCPR Publication No. 99-0050. Rockville, MD: Agency for Health Care Policy and Research.

19   As above.

20   Finkel M F (1997) **The diagnosis and treatment of the adult attention deficit hyperactivity disorders**. *Neurologist*, **3**, 31–44.

by Professor Peter Hill

What developments have there been in the management of attention-deficit hyperactivity disorder?

In terms of treatment, the major development has been the huge MTA trial, now reporting in a number of papers.[21] Although the major finding was that there was no superiority for combined behavioural and medication interventions over carefully titrated medication alone, criticisms have been made that the behavioural (psychosocial) intervention was not of sufficient duration to allow a fair comparison to be made.

There has been considerable interest in the issue of comorbidity[22] and the implications this has for combinations of treatments. ADHD is typically comorbid, at least in a clinical setting.

Evidence for a genetic basis continues to accumulate. There may well be more than one mechanism since ADHD, as currently defined, is a behavioural syndrome with various causal pathways. There is a contribution from the environment, although this is of secondary importance in most cases.

What are the key messages from new research that are not being widely used?

One message is being intentionally ignored. The National Institute of Clinical Excellence (NICE) has recommended that psychological interventions be tried first, before medication, in spite of a lack of evidence that they are superior to indifferently supervised medication ('community treatment' in the MTA trial, meaning methylphenidate 10 mg twice daily in most instances). This is probably sound advice even though it is based on reasoning rather than findings.

Stimulant medication is often still being given twice a day, yet a regime of three or more doses gives better coverage.

Clonidine is being relatively neglected, although only a minority of cases are likely to benefit from it, usually as supplementary to stimulants rather than as a treatment on its own.

Bupropion is relatively underused, although the evidence from randomised controlled trials (RCTs) is not new.[23]

The persistence of ADHD symptoms into adult life is frequently overlooked by adult psychiatric services. It is still very difficult to hand adolescent cases on to adult services when they leave school.

---

21 See vol. 28, issue 6 of the *Journal of Abnormal Child Psychology*. See also vol. 20, issue 2 of the *Journal of the American Academy of Child and Adolescent Psychiatry*, which contains several papers on the MTA study.

22 See e.g. Brown T E (ed.) (2000) **Attention-Deficit Disorders and Comorbidities in Children, Adolescents and Adults**. Washington DC/London: APA.

23 See e.g. Barrickman L, Perry, P J, Allen, A J, *et al* (1995) *Journal of the American Academy of Child and Adolescent Psychiatry*, **34**, 649–657; Conners C K, Casat, C D, Gaultieri, C T, *et al* (1996) *Journal of the American Academy of Child and Adolescent Psychiatry*, **35**, 1314–1321.

REFERENCES

● CLINICAL EVIDENCE ●

Joughin C, Zwi M & Ramchandani P (2001) **Treatment of children with attention deficit hyperactivity disorder (ADHD)**. In *Clinical Evidence: A Compendium of the Best Available Evidence for Effective Health Care*, Issue 5, pp. 205–213. London: BMJ Publishing Group.

● SYSTEMATIC REVIEWS AND META-ANALYSES ●

Baer R A & Nietzel M T (1991) **Cognitive and behavioral treatment of impulsivity in children: A meta-analytic review of the outcome literature**. *Journal of Clinical Child Psychology*, **20**, 400–412.

Connor D F, Fletcher K E & Swanson J M (1999) **A meta-analysis of clonidine for symptoms of attention-deficit hyperactivity disorder**. *Journal of the American Academy of Child and Adolescent Psychiatry*, **38**, 1551–1559.

Corkum P, Tannock R & Moldofsky H (1998) **Sleep disturbances in children with attention-deficit/hyperactivity disorder**. *Journal of the American Academy of Child and Adolescent Psychiatry*, **37**, 637–646.

DuPaul G J & Eckert T L (1997) **The effects of school-based interventions for attention deficit hyperactivity disorder: A meta-analysis**. *School Psychology Review*, **26**, 5–27.

Faraone S, Faraone V & Biederman J (1994) **Is attention deficit hyperactivity disorder familial?** *Harvard Review of Psychiatry*, **1**, 271–287.

Gaub M & Carlson C L (1997) **Gender differences in ADHD: A meta-analysis and critical review**. *Journal of the American Academy of Child and Adolescent Psychiatry*, **36**, 1036–1045.

—— & —— (1997) **Gender differences in ADHD: A meta-analysis and critical review: Erratum**. *Journal of the American Academy of Child and Adolescent Psychiatry*, **36**, 1783.

Green M, Wong M, Atkins D, *et al* (1999) *Diagnosis of Attention Deficit/Hyperactivity Disorder*. Technical Review No. 3 (prepared by Technical Resources International, Inc. under contract no. 290-94-2024). AHCPR publication no. 99-0050. Rockville, MD: Agency for Health Care and Policy Research.

Jadad A R, Booker L, Gauld M, *et al* (1999) **The treatment of attention-deficit hyperactivity disorder: an annotated bibliography and critical appraisal of published systematic reviews and metaanalyses**. *Canadian Journal of Psychiatry*, **44**, 1025–1035.

Kavale K (1982) **The efficacy of stimulant drug treatment for hyperactivity: a meta-analysis**. *Journal of Learning Disabilities*, **15**, 280–289.

—— & Forness S R (1983) **Hyperactivity and diet treatment: a meta-analysis of the Feingold hypothesis**. *Journal of Learning Disabilities*, **16**, 324–330.

Klassen A, Miller A, Raina P, *et al* (1999) **Attention-deficit hyperactivity disorder in children and youth: a quantitative systematic review of the**

efficacy of different management strategies. *Canadian Journal of Psychiatry*, **44**, 1007–1016.

Losier B J, McGrath P J & Klein R M (1996) **Error patterns of the Continuous Performance Test in non-medicated and medicated samples of children with and without ADHD: A meta-analytic review**. *Journal of Child Psychology and Psychiatry and Allied Disciplines*, **37**, 971–987.

Miller A, Lee S, Raina P, *et al* (1998) *A Review of Therapies for Attention-Deficit/Hyperactivity Disorder*. Ottawa: Canadian Co-ordinating Office for Health Technology Assessment (CCOHTA).

Silva R R, Munoz D M & Alpert M (1996) **Carbamazepine use in children and adolescents with features of attention-deficit hyperactivity disorder: A meta-analysis**. *Journal of the American Academy of Child and Adolescent Psychiatry*, **35**, 352–358.

Stein M A, Krasowski M, Leventhal B L, *et al* (1996) **Behavioral and cognitive effects of methylzanthines: a meta-analysis of theophylline and caffeine**. *Archives of Pediatrics and Adolescent Medicine*, **150**, 284–288.

Swanson J M, Cantwell D, Lerner M, *et al* (1993) **Effects of stimulant medication on learning in children with ADHD**. *Exceptional Children*, **60**, 154–161.

Thurber S & Walker C E (1983) **Medication and hyperactivity: a meta-analysis**. *Journal of General Psychology*, **108**, 79–86.

● PRACTICE PARAMETERS ●

American Academy of Child and Adolescent Psychiatry (1997) **Practice parameters for the assessment and treatment of children, adolescents and adults with attention deficit hyperactivity disorder**. *Journal of the American Academy of Child Adolescent Psychiatry*, **36** (suppl.), 85S–121S.

● CLINICAL GUIDELINES ●

Taylor E, Sergeant J & Doepfner M (1998) **European guidelines: clinical guidelines for ADHD**. *Journal of European Child and Adolescent Psychiatry*, **7**, 184–200.

● REVIEWS ●

Hill P (1998) **Attention-deficit hyperactivity disorder**. *Archives of Disease in Childhood*, **79**, 381–384.

—— & Taylor E (2001) **An auditable protocol for treating attention deficit/hyperactivity disorder**. *Archives of Disease in Childhood*, **84**, 404–409.

Overmeyer S & Taylor E (1999) **Annotation: principles of treatment for hyperkinetic disorder: practical approaches for the UK**. *Journal of Child Psychology and Psychiatry*, **40**, 1147–1157.

Pliszka S R, Greenhill L L, Crismon M L, *et al* (2000) **The Texas children's medication algorithm project: Report of the Texas consensus conference panel on medication of childhood attention-deficit/hyperactivity disorder. Parts I and II**. *Journal of the American Academy of Child and Adolescent Psychiatry*, **39**, 908–919, 920–927.

● CLASSIC PAPERS ●

Bradley C (1937) **The behaviour of children receiving benzedrine**. *American Journal of Orthopsychiatry*, **15**, 577–585.

● CUTTING EDGE PAPERS ●

The MTA Cooperative Group (1999) **A 14-month randomised clinical trial of treatment strategies for attention-deficit/hyperactivity disorder**. *Archives of General Psychiatry*, **56**, 1073–1086.

Sunohara G A, Roberts W, Malone M, *et al* (2000) **Linkage of the dopamine D4 receptor gene and attention-deficit/hyperactivity disorder**. *Journal of the American Academy of Child and Adolescent Psychiatry*, **39**, 1537–1542.

Taylor E (1999) **Developmental neuropsychopathology of attention deficit and impulsiveness**. In *Development and Psychopathology*, **11**, 607–628.

Thapar A, Holmes J, Poulton K, *et al* (1999) **Genetic basis of attention deficit and hyperactivity**. *British Journal of Psychiatry*, **174**, 105–111.

Wells K C, Pelham W E, Kotkin R A, *et al* (2000) **Psychosocial treatment strategies in the MTA study: Rationale, methods, and critical issues in design and implementation**. *Journal of Abnormal Child Psychology*, **28**, 483–505.

● REPORTS ●

Gilmore A, Best L & Milne R (1998) *Methylphenidate in Children with Hyperactivity*. DEC Report 78. Bristol: South and West Research and Development Directorate.

National Institute of Clinical Excellence (2000) *Guidance on the Use of Methylphenidate (Ritalin, Equasym) for Attention Deficit/Hyperactivity Disorder in Childhood*. Technology Appraisal Guidance – No. 13. London: National Institute of Clinical Excellence.

● FOCUS REPORTS ●

Joughin C & Zwi M (1999) *FOCUS on the Use of Stimulants in Children with Attention Deficit Hyperactivity Disorder: A Primary Evidence-Base Briefing*. London: Royal College of Psychiatrists' Research Unit. (Presently being updated.)

● USEFUL WEBSITES ●

ADDNet UK http://www.btinternet.com/~black.ice/addnet

Children and Adolescents with Attention Deficit/Hyperactivity Disorder (CHADD) http://www.chadd.org

Mental Health Foundation http://www.mentalhealth.org.uk

Mind http://www.mind.org.uk

Cochrane Controlled Trials Register

187 hits (keywords: ADHD AND child*)

493 hits (keywords: "attention deficit hyperactivity disorder" AND child*)

Cochrane Developmental, Psychosocial and Learning Problems Group
Contact: Dr Jane Dennis, Bristol, UK. J.Dennis@bristol.ac.uk

BULLYING

INTRODUCTION

Bullying is the intentional, unprovoked abuse of power by one or more children to inflict pain or cause distress to another child on repeated occasions. It is particularly likely to occur in social groups with clear power relationships and low supervision. It occurs to some extent in all schools and often without apparent provocation. Bullying is more common in boys and in the youngest pupils in a school. The commonest type of bullying is general name calling, followed by physically hitting someone, issuing of threats and the spreading of rumours about someone.

Research suggests an incidence of about 1 in 5 for being bullied and up to 1 in 10 for bullying others[24] (with higher figures being quoted for children who attend remedial classes[25] or who are of Asian origin).[26]

REFERENCES

● SYSTEMATIC REVIEWS AND META-ANALYSES ●

Hawker D S J & Boulton M J (2000) **Twenty years' research on peer victimization and psychosocial maladjustment: A meta-analytic review of cross sectional studies**. *Journal of Child Psychology and Psychiatry*, **41**, 441–455.

Mytton J & DiGuiseppi C (2000) *School based prevention programmes for reducing violence*. Protocol for Cochrane Review. In *The Cochrane Library*, Issue 4. Oxford: Update Software.

● REVIEWS ●

Salmon G & West A (2000) **Physical and mental health issues related to bullying in schools**. *Current Opinion in Psychiatry*, **13**, 375–380.

——, James A, Cassidy E C, *et al* (2000) **Bullying: a review. Presentations to an adolescent psychiatric service and within a school for emotionally and behaviourally disturbed children**. *Clinical Child Psychology and Psychiatry*, **5**, 563–579.

● CLASSIC PAPERS ●

Dawkins J (1995) **Bullying in schools: doctors' responsibilities**. *British Medical Journal*, **310**, 274–275.

Olweus D (1994) **Annotation: Bullying at school: basic facts and effects of a school based intervention program**. *Journal of Child Psychology and Psychiatry*, **7**, 1171–1190.

24   Whitney I & Smith P K (1993) **A survey of the nature and extent of bullying in junior/middle and secondary schools**. *Educational Research*, **35**, 3–25.
25   Moran S, Smith P K, Thompson D, *et al* (1993) **Ethnic differences in experiences of bullying: Asian and white children**. *British Journal of Educational Psychology*, **63**, 431–440.
26   O'Moore A M & Hillery B (1989) **Bullying in Dublin schools**. *Irish Journal of Psychology*, **10**, 426–441.

Slee P T (1994) **Situational and interpersonal correlates of anxiety associated with peer victimization**. *Child Psychiatry and Human Development*, **25**, 97–107.

Whitney I & Smith P K (1993) **A survey of the nature and extent of bullying in junior/middle and secondary schools**. *Education Research*, **35**, 3–25.

Williams K, Chambers M, Logan S, *et al* (1996) **Association of common health symptoms with bullying in primary school children**. *British Medical Journal*, **313**, 17–19.

● CUTTING EDGE PAPERS ●

Kumpulainen K, Rasanen E, Henttonem I, *et al* (1998) **Bullying and psychiatric symptoms among elementary school-age children**. *Child Abuse and Neglect*, **22**, 705–717.

—, — & — (1999) **Children involved in bullying: Psychological disturbance and the persistence of the involvement**. *Child Abuse and Neglect*, **23**, 1253–1262.

Rigby K (1999) **Peer victimization at school and the health of secondary school students**. *British Journal of Educational Psychology*, **69**, 95–104.

— & Slee P (1999) **Suicidal ideation among adolescent school children, involvement in bully-victim problems and perceived social support**. *Suicide and Life-Threatening Behaviour*, **29**, 119–130.

Salmon G, James A & Smith D M (1998) **Bullying in schools: self reported anxiety, depression and self esteem in secondary school children**. *British Medical Journal*, **317**, 924–925.

Smith P K & Myron-Wilson R (1998) **Parenting and school bullying**. *Clinical Child Psychology and Psychiatry*, **3**, 405–417.

— & Shu S (2000) **What good schools can do about bullying: Findings from a survey in English schools after a decade of research and action**. *Childhood*, **8**, 193–212.

Sutton J, Smith P K & Swettenham J (1999) **Social cognition and bullying: Social inadequacy or skilled manipulation?** *British Journal of Development Psychology*, **17**, 435–450.

● BOOKS ●

Olweus D (1993) ***Bullying in Schools: What we know and what we can do***. Oxford: Blackwell.

Rigby K (1996) ***Bullying in Schools and what to do about it***. London: Jessica Kingsley.

Skinner A (1996) ***Bullying: An Annotated Bibliography of Literature and Resources***. 2nd edn. Leicester: Youth Work Press.

Smith P K & Sharp S (eds) (1994) ***School Bullying: Insights and Perspectives***. London: Routledge.

—, Morita Y, Junger-Tas J, *et al* (eds) (1999) ***The Nature of School Bullying: A Cross National Perspective***. New York and London: Routledge.

Tattum D P & Lane D A (eds) (1989) ***Bullying in Schools***. Stoke-on-Trent: Trentham Books.

Bullying on-line http:// www.bullying.co.uk

Cochrane Controlled Trials Register
1 hit (keywords: bully*)

Cochrane Developmental, Psychosocial and Learning Problems Group
Contact: Dr Jane Dennis, Bristol, UK. J.Dennis@bristol.ac.uk

CONDUCT DISORDERS AND JUVENILE DELINQUENCY

INTRODUCTION

Conduct disorders are characterised by a repetitive and persistent pattern of dissocial, aggressive or defiant conduct. Examples of the behaviours on which the diagnosis is based include the following: excessive levels of fighting or bullying; cruelty to animals or other people; severe destructiveness to property; fire-setting; stealing; repeated lying; truancy from school and running away from home; unusually frequent and severe temper tantrums; defiant provocative behaviour; and persistent severe disobedience. Such behaviour, when at its most extreme for the individual, should amount to major violations of age-appropriate social expectations, and is therefore more severe than ordinary childish mischief or adolescent rebelliousness. Isolated dissocial or criminal acts are not in themselves grounds for the diagnosis, which implies an enduring pattern of behaviour of at least six months.[27]

Juvenile delinquency is a legal term for children with antisocial behaviour who are involved in breaking the law.[28]

Conduct disorders are the most frequently diagnosed disorders for children.[29] The 1999 Office of National Statistics survey of the mental health of 5–15-year-old children reported the prevalence of conduct disorders to be 7.4% of boys and 3.2% of girls in Great Britain. The rates of disorder were higher in poorer areas, in lone-parent families, and in unemployed households.[30] The prevalence of conduct disorders in Western countries has increased five-fold over the past 70 years.[31]

Conduct disorders in childhood predicts many adverse developmental outcomes, including educational underachievement, juvenile offending, substance misuse and dependence, anxiety, depression and suicide attempts. Among children with conduct disorder, 25–40% will go on to develop dissocial personality disorder in adult life. Dissocial personality is itself associated with elevated rates of mortality, offending behaviour, marital disharmony, mental health problems, and, most importantly for the intergenerational transmission of the disorder, children with conduct disorder.

DIAGNOSIS

The ICD–10 includes six categories for the diagnosis of conduct disorder:

- ○ Conduct disorder confined to the family context: there is no significant conduct disturbance outside the family, and the child's social relationships outside the family are normal.

- ○ Unsocialised conduct disorder: associated with disturbed peer relationships characterised by isolation, rejection and lack of lasting, empathic, reciprocal relationships with peers.

27 World Health Organization (1992) *The ICD–10 Classification of Mental and Behavioural Disorders. Clinical Descriptions and Diagnostic Guidelines*. Geneva: WHO.

28 Berelowitz M & Nelki J (1993) **Clinical syndromes in middle childhood**. In *Seminars in Child and Adolescent Psychiatry* (eds D Black & D Cottrell). London: Gaskell.

29 American Psychiatric Association (2000) *Diagnostic and Statistical Manual of Mental Disorders*. 4th edn (DSM–IV–TR). Washington DC: APA.

30 Meltzer H, Gatward R, Goodman R, *et al* (2000) *The Mental Health of Children and Adolescents in Great Britain*. London: The Stationery Office.

31 Robins L N (1999) **A 70-year history of conduct disorder: Variations in definition, prevalence, and correlates**. In *Historical and Geographical Influences on Psychopathology* (ed. P Cohen), pp. 37–56. Mahwah, NJ: Lawrence Erlbaum Associates.

- ○ Socialised conduct disorder: associated with adequate lasting relationships with peers who are usually, but not necessarily, other young people involved in delinquent or dissocial activities.

- ○ Oppositional defiant disorder (ODD): usually seen in children under the age of 9 or 10 years and excludes any form of severe dissocial behaviour in violation of the law or rights of others. Regarded by many authorities as a less severe type of, or developmental antecedent to, conduct disorder.

- ○ Other conduct disorders and conduct disorder, unspecified.

The DSM–IV bases the diagnosis of conduct disorder on the presence of specific diagnostic criteria under the headings of aggression to people and animals (seven criteria), destruction of property (two criteria), deceitfulness or theft (three criteria), and serious violations of rules (three criteria). In order to qualify, three or more criteria must be present for 12 months and at least one for six months. Subtypes of conduct disorder are based upon age of onset of the disorder and can occur in mild, moderate and severe forms. The three subtypes are:

- ○ childhood-onset type: onset of at least one criterion characteristic of conduct disorder prior to the age of 10 years. The behaviour tends to be characterised by disturbed peer relations, and is therefore closely related to ICD–10 unsocialised conduct disorder;

- ○ adolescent-onset type: symptoms of conduct disorder were not present before the age of 10 years. The behaviour is usually characterised by normal peer relations, and is therefore closely related to ICD–10 socialised conduct disorder; and

- ○ unspecified onset.

Oppositional defiant disorder is regarded as a completely separate diagnostic category in the DSM–IV system. A further category of 'Disruptive behaviour not otherwise specified' is available for those not meeting strict criteria for conduct disorder or ODD.

AETIOLOGY

The development of conduct disorders appears to be associated predominantly with disadvantaged backgrounds, but can be best understood in terms of a risk-resilience model. The progressive accumulation of risk factors across development, in association with the absence of protective factors, leads to an increased likelihood that conduct disorder will develop.[32]

The major risk factors are:

- ○ genetic: males are more likely to suffer from conduct disorders than females. Other genetic factors require the presence of environmental risk for their expression;

- ○ difficult temperament with poor emotional regulation;

- ○ neurodevelopmental and cognitive problems: hyperactivity executive function deficits, language delay, lowered intelligence, social information processing showing hostile attributional bias; and

---

32 Farrington D P (1999) **Conduct disorder and delinquency**. In *Risks and Outcomes in Developmental Psychopathology* (eds H C Steinhausen & F C Verhulst), pp.165–192. Oxford: OUP.

○ environmental risk: poverty and unemployment, smoking in pregnancy, parental psychopathology (especially maternal depression and paternal antisocial personality disorder), parental alcohol or substance misuse, parental discord, poor parenting, insecure attachment, teacher and peer rejection, delinquent peer affiliation, early onset of youth drug and alcohol misuse.

The major protective factors are: easy temperament, high IQ, secure attachment and positive parenting, at least one positive relationship with an adult, positive school and community ethos promoting pro-social behaviour, participation in positive recreational activities, and association with non-delinquent peers.

CRITICAL QUESTIONS

by Dr Julian Morrell

What are the new developments in the understanding and management of conduct disorders?

There are multiple contextual levels of influence in conduct disorder such as: cultural factors; the social construction of antisocial behaviour; the community and family contexts within which antisocial behaviour occurs; and how the above factors interact with individual biological, genetic and cognitive factors throughout childhood and across the life course. Conduct disorder can now be comprehensively researched using new statistical techniques of multilevel modelling in longitudinal research designs.[33]

Research into the role of parenting quality in infancy for the development of self-regulatory capacity has shown that the development of emotional dysregulation in the context of emotionally rejecting parenting and maternal depression predicts subsequent conduct disorder, especially in boys.[34] In addition, early trauma leads to dysregulation of the hypothalamo–pituitary–adrenal axis and associated problems with the regulation of arousal and aggressive behaviour.[35] This evidence, together with prevention studies showing benefit, especially if intervention occurs in infancy[36] or the preschool period,[37] supports the strategy of early intervention to prevent conduct disorder.

Robust evidence exists for the efficacy of behavioural parenting training programmes[38] for children with conduct disorder aged three years and upwards. For children aged

33 Boyle M H & Willms J D (2001) Multilevel modelling of hierarchical data in developmental studies. *Journal of Child Psychology and Psychiatry*, **42**, 141–162.

34 Raine A, Brennan P & Mednick S A (1994) Birth complications combined with early maternal rejection at age 1 year predispose to violent crime at age 18 years. *Archives of General Psychiatry*, **51**, 984–988; Shaw D S, Winslow E B, Owens E B, *et al* (1998) The development of early externalizing problems among children from low-income families: A transformational perspective. *Journal of Abnormal Child Psychology*, **26**, 95–107.

35 McBurnett, K, Lahey B B, Rathauz P J, *et al* (2000) Low salivary cortisol and persistent aggression in boys referred for disruptive behavior. *Archives of General Psychiatry*, **57**, 38–43.

36 van den Boom D C (1995) Do first-year intervention effects endure? Follow-up during toddlerhood of a sample of Dutch irritable infants. *Child Development*, **66**, 1798–1816.

37 Berrueta-Clement J R, Schweinhart L J, *et al* (1987) The effects of early educational intervention on crime and delinquency in adolescence and early adulthood. Prevention of delinquent behavior. In *Vermont Conference on the Primary Prevention of Psychopathology*, Vol. 10 (eds J D Burchard & S N Burchard), pp. 220–240. Beverly Hills, CA: Sage Publications.

38 Barlow J (1999) *Systematic Review of the Effectiveness of Parent Training Programmes in Improving Behavioural Problems in Children Aged 3–10 Years*. Oxford: Department of Public Health, Health Services Research Unit.

five years and above, the combination of parent training and child problem-solving skills training may confer additional benefit.[39]

Good evidence exists for efficacy of multi-systemic therapy in severely disturbed children and adolescents with conduct disorder.[40]

Research also suggests that school-based behavioural interventions can be effective, especially for very severely disturbed children.[41]

Evidence exists showing that, in severely disturbed conduct disordered youths with chronic offending histories, 'Treatment Foster Care' is more effective than group residential care.[42]

There is some weak evidence for efficacy of risperidone and lithium in the treatment of highly aggressive hospitalised children with conduct disorder, but the sample sizes in these RCTs were very low, and lithium, in particular, was very poorly tolerated.[43]

What are the key messages from new research that are not being widely used?

Parent training programmes are not widely available and recruitment strategies need to be more proactive for these interventions, where available, to be fully successful.

Multi-systemic therapy is most suitable for severe cases, however it is not widely available. Moreover, conventional out-patient child psychiatric treatment is often not suitable for youths with severe conduct disorder, as the level of need is too high; neither is in-patient treatment, as their behaviour proves too disruptive. Hence, such youths often do not receive adequate service provision.[44] A strong case can therefore be made that each area should possess a 'multi-disciplinary severe conduct disorder team' adhering to the principles of multi-systemic therapy, and where necessary using Treatment Foster Care, to address the complex multi-dimensional problems of these youths.

School-based interventions are not widely available. Indeed, the policy of exclusion increases the chances of delinquent peer affiliation and further deviant development.

Treatment Foster Care as such does not exist in the UK, the closest approximation being foster care plus placements. However, the numbers of available foster parents, and the level of training and support offered to foster parents is inadequate.

Early intervention to support parenting in infancy and the pre-school years is also not widely available. Although government initiatives such as Surestart aim to provide such services, a commitment of these services to evidence-based practice along the lines of

39 Webster-Stratton C (1993) **Strategies for helping early school-aged children with oppositional defiant and conduct disorders: the importance of home–school partnerships.** *School Psychology Review*, **22**, 437–457.

40 Henggeler S W (1999) **Multisystemic therapy: An overview of clinical procedures, outcomes, and policy implications.** *Child Psychology and Psychiatry Review*, **4**, 2–10.

41 Stoolmiller M, Eddy J M & Reid J B (2000) **Detecting and describing preventive intervention effects in a universal school-based randomized trial targeting delinquent and violent behaviour.** *Journal of Consulting and Clinical Psychology*, **68**, 296–306.

42 Chamberlain P & Moore K (1998) **A clinical model for parenting juvenile offenders: A comparison of group care versus family care.** *Clinical Child Psychology and Psychiatry*, **3**, 375–386.

43 Findling R L, McNamara N K, Branicky L A, *et al* (2000) **A double-blind pilot study of risperidone in the treatment of conduct disorder.** *Journal of the American Academy of Child and Adolescent Psychiatry*, **39**, 509–516; Malone R P, Delaney M A, Leubbert J F, *et al* (2000) **A double-blind placebo-controlled study of lithium in hospitalized aggressive children and adolescents with conduct disorder.** *Archives of General Psychiatry*, **57**, 649–654.

44 Street C (2000) *Whose Crisis? Meeting the Needs of Children and Young People with Serious Mental Health Problems.* London: Young Minds.

promoting maternal sensitivity to infant cues[45] is needed. In addition, perinatal and infant psychiatry services are not widely available or coordinated, reducing the availability of effective mother–infant care for those suffering from severe postnatal depression.

Children with conduct disorder are still being offered both group therapy, which has been shown to be harmful, and supportive counselling, which is often ineffective.

REFERENCES

● SYSTEMATIC REVIEWS AND META-ANALYSES ●

Andrews D A, Bonta J & Hoge R D (1990) **Classification for effective rehabilitation**. *Criminal Justice and Behavior*, **17**, 19–51.

Antonowitcz D & Ross R R (1994) **Essential components of successful rehabilitation programs for offenders**. *International Journal of Offender Therapy and Comparative Criminology*, **38**, 97–104.

Arbuthnot J & Gordon D A (1988) **Crime and cognition: Community applications of sociomoral reasoning development**. *Criminal Justice and Behavior*, **15**, 379–393.

Baer R A & Nietzel M T (1991) **Cognitive and behavioral treatment of impulsivity in children: A meta-analytic review of the outcome literature**. *Journal of Clinical Child Psychology*, **20**, 400–412.

Barlow J (1999) *Systematic Review of the Effectiveness of Parent Training Programmes in Improving Behavioural Problems in Children Aged 3–10 Years*. Oxford: Department of Public Health, Health Services Research Unit.

Bender W N & Smith J K (1990) **Classroom behavior of children and adolescents with learning disabilities: a meta-analysis**. *Journal of Learning Disability*, **23**, 298–305.

Bennett D S & Gibbons T A (2000) **Efficacy of child cognitive-behavioral interventions for antisocial behavior: A meta-analysis**. *Child and Family Behavior Therapy*, **22**, 1–15.

Casey P & Keilitz I (1990) **Estimating the prevalence of learning disabled and mentally retarded juvenile offenders: A meta-analysis**. In *Understanding Troubled and Troubling Youth* (ed. P E Leone), pp. 82–101. Thousand Oaks, CA: Sage Publications.

Durlak J A, Fuhrman T & Lampman C (1991) **Effectiveness of cognitive– behavior therapy for maladapting children: A meta-analysis**. *Psychological Bulletin*, **110**, 204–214.

Dush D M, Hirt M L & Schroeder H E (1989) **Self statement modification in the treatment of child behaviour disorders: a meta-analysis**. *Psychological Bulletin*, **106**, 97–106.

Frick P J, Lahey B B, Loeber R, *et al* (1993) **Oppositional defiant disorder and conduct disorder: a meta-analytic review of factor analyses and cross-validation in a clinic sample**. *Clinical Psychology Review*, **13**, 319–340.

---

45   van den Boom D C (1995) Do first-year intervention effects endure? Follow-up during toddlerhood of a sample of Dutch irritable infants. *Child Development*, **66**, 1798–1816.

Garrett P (1985) **Effects of residential treatment of adjudicated delinquents: A meta-analysis**. *Journal of Research in Crime and Delinquency*, **22**, 287–308.

Gensheimer L K, Mayer J P, Gottschalk R, *et al* (1986) **Diverting youth from the juvenile justice system: A meta-analysis of intervention efficacy**. In *Youth Violence: Programmes and Prospects* (eds S J Apter & A Goldstein), pp. 39–57. Elmsford, NY: Pergamon Press.

Gottschalk R, Davidson W S I, Gensheimer L K, *et al* (1987) **Community-based interventions**. In *Handbook of Juvenile Delinquency* (ed. H Quay), pp. 266–289. New York: John Wiley & Sons.

—, —, Mayer J, *et al* (1987) **Behavioral approaches with juvenile offenders: A meta-analysis of long-term treatment efficacy**. In *Behavioral Approaches to Crime and Delinquency* (eds E Morris & C J Braukmann), pp. 399–422. New York: Plenum Press.

Griffiths M (1999) **Violent video games and aggression: a review of the literature**. *Aggression and Violent Behaviour*, **4**, 203–212.

Izzo R L & Ross R R (1990) **Meta-analysis of rehabilitation programs for juvenile delinquents: A brief report**. *Criminal Justice and Behavior*, **17**, 134–142.

Joiner T E & Wagner K D (1996) **Parental, child-centered attributions and outcome: A meta-analytic review with conceptual and methodological implications**. *Journal of Abnormal Child Psychology*, **24**, 37–52.

Kaufman P (1995) **Meta-analysis of juvenile delinquency prevention programs.** Unpublished Master's thesis. Reported in Lipsey M W (1988) **Juvenile delinquency interventions**. In *Lessons from Selected Program and Policy Areas. New Directions for Program Evaluation* (eds H S Bloom, D S Cordray, *et al*), pp. 63–84. San Francisco, CA: Jossey-Bass.

Kavale K A, Mathur S R, Forness S R, *et al* (1997) **Effectiveness of social skills training for students with behaviour disorders: a meta-analysis**. *Advances in Learning and Behavioural Disabilities*, **11**, 1–26.

Lipsey M (1992) **Juvenile deliquency treatment: a meta-analytic inquiry into the variability of effects**. In *Meta-Analysis for Explanation: A Casebook* (eds T D Cook, H Cooper, D S Cordray, *et al*), pp. 83–128. Thousand Oaks, CA: Russell Sage Foundation.

— (1992) **The effect of treatment on juvenile delinquents: Results from meta-analysis**. In *Social Intervention: Potential and Constraints* (eds F Loesel, B Bender & T Bliesener), pp. 131–143. Berlin: Walter De Gruyter.

Loeber R & Schmaling K B (1985) **Empirical evidence for overt and covert patterns of antisocial conduct problems: a meta-analysis**. *Journal of Abnormal Child Psychology*, **13**, 337–353.

— & Stouthamer-Loeber M (1986) **Family factors as correlates and predictors of juvenile conduct problems and delinquency: a meta-analysis**. In *Crime and Justice Annual Review of Research* (eds M Ronry & N Moris), pp. 29–149. Chicago, IL: University of Chicago.

Losel F (1987) **Psychological crime prevention: Concepts, evaluations and perspectives**. In *Social Intervention: Potential and Constraints* (eds G Albrecht & H U Otto), pp. 289–313. Berlin/New York: Walter de Gruyter.

Losel F & Koferl P (1989) **Evaluation research on correctional treatment in West Germany: A meta-analysis**. In *Criminal Behavior and the Justice System:*

Psychological Perspectives (eds H Wegener, F Losel & J Haisch), pp. 334–355. New York: Springer.

Mayer J P, Gensheimer L K, Davidson W S I, *et al* (1986) **Social learning treatment within juvenile justice: A meta-analysis of impact in the natural environment**. In *Youth Violence: Programmes and Prospects* (eds S J Apter & A Goldstein), pp. 24–38. Elmsford, NY: Pergamon Press.

Miller P A & Eisenberg N (1988) **The relation of empathy to aggressive and externalizing/antisocial behaviour**. *Psychological Bulletin*, **103**, 324–344.

Montogomery P (2001) **Media-based behavioural treatments for behavioural disorders in children**. Protocol for Cochrane Review. In *The Cochrane Library*, Issue 1. Oxford: Update Software.

Mytton J & Di Guiseppi C (2001) **School based prevention programmes for reducing violence**. Protocol for Cochrane Review. In *The Cochrane Library*, Issue 1. Oxford: Update Software.

Nelson J R, Smith D J & Dodd J (1990) **The moral reasoning of juvenile delinquents: A meta-analysis**. *Journal of Abnormal Child Psychology*, **18**, 231–239.

Oosterlaan J, Logan G D & Sergeant J A (1998) **Response inhibition in AD/HD, CD, comorbid AD/HD + CD, anxious, and control children: a meta-analysis of studies with the stop task**. *Journal of Child Psychology and Psychiatry and Allied Disciplines*, **39**, 411–425.

Redondo S, Sanchez-Meca J & Garrido V (1999) **The influence of treatment programmes on the recidivism of juvenile and adult offenders: A European meta-analytic review**. *Psychology, Crime and Law*, **5**, 251–278.

Serketich W J & Dumas J E (1996) **The effectiveness of behavioural parent training to modify antisocial behaviour in children: a meta-analysis**. *Behaviour Therapy*, **27**, 171–186.

Weaver T L & Clum G A (1995) **Psychological distress associated with interpersonal violence: a meta-analysis**. *Clinical Psychology Review*, **15**, 115–140.

Wells L E & Rankin J H (1991) **Families and delinquency: A meta-analysis of the impact of broken homes**. *Social Problems*, **38**, 71–93.

Whitehead J T & Lab S P (1989) **A meta-analysis of juvenile correctional treatment**. *Journal of Research in Crime and Delinquency*, **26**, 276–295.

Wilson S J & Lipsey M W (2000) **Wilderness challenge programs for delinquent youth: A meta-analysis of outcome evaluations**. *Evaluation and Program Planning*, **23**, 1–12.

Woodward M, Williams P, Nursten J, *et al* (1999) **The epidemiology of mentally disordered offending: a systematic review of studies, based in the general population, of criminality combined with psychiatric illness**. *Journal of Epidemiology and Biostatistics*, **4**, 101–113.

Woolfenden S, Williams K & Peat J (2001) **Family parenting interventions for conduct disorder and delinquency in children aged 10–17**. Cochrane Review. In *The Cochrane Library*, Issue 1. Oxford: Update Software.

Zoccolillo M (1992) **Co-occurrence of conduct disorder and its adult outcomes with depressive and anxiety disorders: a review**. *Journal of the American Academy of Child and Adolescent Psychiatry*, **31**, 547–556.

● PRACTICE PARAMETERS ●

American Academy of Child and Adolescent Psychiatry (1997) **Practice Parameters for the assessment and treatment of children and adolescents with conduct disorder**. *Journal of the American Academy of Child and Adolescent Psychiatry*, **36** (suppl.), 122–139.

● REVIEWS ●

Alexander J F, Holtzworth-Munroe A & Jameson P B (1994) **The process and outcome of marital and family therapy: Research review and evaluation**. In *Handbook of Psychotherapy and Behavior Change* (eds A E Bergin & S L Garfield), pp. 595–630. 4th edn. New York: John Wiley & Sons.

Ben-Amos B (1992) **Depression and conduct disorders in children and adolescents: A review of the literature**. *Bulletin of the Menninger Clinic*, **56**, 188–208.

Brennan P A & Raine A (1997) **Biosocial bases of antisocial behavior: Psychophysiological, neurological, and cognitive factors**. *Clinical Psychology Review*, **17**, 589–604.

Bryant D, Vizzard L H, Willoughby M, *et al* (1999) **A review of interventions for preschoolers with aggressive and disruptive behavior**. *Early Education and Development*, **10**, 47–68.

Campbell M & Cueva J E (1995) **Psychopharmacology in child and adolescent psychiatry: a review of the past seven years. Part II**. *Journal of the American Academy of Child and Adolescent Psychiatry*, **34**, 1262–1272.

Crick N R & Dodge K A (1994) **A review and reformulation of social information-processing mechanisms in children's social adjustment**. *Psychological Bulletin*, **115**, 74–101.

Drewett A & Shepperdson B (1995) *A Literature Review of Services for Mentally Disordered Offenders*. Leicester: Nuffield Community Care Studies Unit.

Eme R F & Kavanaugh L (1995) **Sex differences in conduct disorder**. *Journal of Clinical Child Psychology*, **24**, 406–426.

Fonagy P & Target M (1994) **The efficacy of psychoanalysis for children with disruptive disorders**. *Journal of the American Academy of Child and Adolescent Psychiatry*, **33**, 45–55.

Foote R, Eyberg S, Schuhmann, E,*et al* (1998) **Parent–child interaction approaches to the treatment of child behavior problems**. *Advances in Clinical Child Psychology*, **20**, 125–152.

Gardner F E (1992) **Parent–child interaction and conduct disorder**. *Educational Psychology Review*, **4**, 135–163.

Greenberg M T, DeKlyen M, Speltz, M L, *et al* (1997) **The role of attachment processes in externalizing psychopathology in young children**. In *Attachment and Psychopathology* (ed. K Zucker *et al*), pp. 196–222. Seattle, WA: Guilford Press.

Greenwood P W (1996) **Responding to juvenile crime: lessons learned**. *Future of Children*, **6**, 75–85.

Henggeler S W (1999) **Multisystemic therapy: An overview of clinical procedures, outcomes, and policy implications**. *Child Psychology and Psychiatry Review*, **4**, 2–10.

Kazdin A E (1997) **Practitioner review: Psychological treatments for conduct disorder in children**. *Journal of Child Psychology and Psychiatry*, **38**, 161–178.

—— (1998) **Current progress and future plans for developing effective treatments: comments and perspectives**. *Journal of Clinical Child Psychology*, **27**, 217–226.

Kendall P C, Reber M, McLeer S, *et al* (1990) **Cognitive-behavioral treatment of conduct-disordered children**. *Cognitive Therapy and Research*, **14**, 379–397.

Loeber R & Farrington D P (1994) **Problems and solutions in longitudinal and experimental treatment studies of child psychopathology and delinquency**. *Journal of Consulting and Clinical Psychology*, **62**, 887–900.

—— & Keenan K (1994) **Interaction between conduct disorder and its comorbid conditions: Effects of age and gender**. *Clinical Psychology Review*, **14**, 497–523.

Maughan B & Rutter M (1998) **Continuities and discontinuities in antisocial behavior from childhood to adult life**. *Advances in Clinical Child Psychology*, **20**, 1–47.

Moffitt T E (1993) **The neuropsychology of conduct disorder**. *Development and Psychopathology*, **5**, 135–151.

Pajer K A (1998) **What happens to 'bad' girls? A review of the adult outcomes of antisocial adolescent girls**. *American Journal of Psychiatry*, **155**, 862–870.

Reddy L A & Pfeiffer S I (1997) **Effectiveness of treatment foster care with children and adolescents: a review of outcome studies**. *Journal of the American Academy of Child and Adolescent Psychiatry*, **36**, 581–588.

Reid J B (1993) **Prevention of conduct disorder before and after school entry: Relating interventions to developmental findings**. *Development and Psychopathology*, **5**, 243–262.

Russo M F & Beidel D C (1994) **Comorbidity of childhood anxiety and externalizing disorders: Prevalence, associated characteristics, and validation issues**. *Clinical Psychology Review*, **14**, 199–221.

Sheldrick C (1999) **Practitioner review: The assessment and management of risk in adolescents**. *Journal of Child Psychology and Psychiatry*, **40**, 507–518.

Snyder H N (1996) **The juvenile court and delinquency cases**. *Future of Children*, **6**, 53–63.

Stewart J T, Myers W C, Burket R C, *et al* (1990) **A review of the pharmaco-therapy of aggression in children and adolescents**. *Journal of the American Academy of Child and Adolescent Psychiatry*, **29**, 269–277.

Templeton J K (1990) **Social skills training for behavior problem adolescents: A review**. *International Journal of Partial Hospitalization*, **6**, 49–60.

Utting D, Bright J & Henricson C (1993) *Crime and The Family*. London: Family Policy Studies Centre.

Webster-Stratton C (1993) **Strategies for helping early school-aged children with oppositional defiant and conduct disorders: the importance of home–school partnerships**. *School Psychology Review*, **22**, 437–457.

—— (1998) **Parent training with low-income families: Promoting parental engagement through a collaborative approach**. In *Handbook of Child Abuse Research and Treatment: Issues in Clinical Child Psychology* (ed. J R Lutzker), pp. 183–210. New York: Plenum Press.

Zoccolillo M (1993) **Gender and the development of conduct disorder**. *Development and Psychopathology*, **5**, 65–78.

Zubieta J K & Alessi N E (1993) **Is there a role of serotonin in the disruptive behavior disorders? A literature review**. *Journal of Child and Adolescent Psychopharmacology*, **3**, 11–35.

● CLASSIC PAPERS ●

Berrueta-Clement J R & Schweinhart L J (1987) **The effects of early educational intervention on crime and delinquency in adolescence and early adulthood. Prevention of delinquent behavior**. In *Vermont Conference on the Primary Prevention of Psychopathology*, Vol. 10 (eds J D Burchard & S N Burchard), pp. 220–240. Beverly Hills, CA: Sage Publications.

Bowlby J (1944) **Forty-four juvenile thieves: their characters and home-life (I)**. *International Journal of Psycho Analysis*, **25**, 19–53.

—— (1944) **Forty-four juvenile thieves: their characters and home-life (II)**. *International Journal of Psycho Analysis*, **25**, 107–128.

Cadoret R J, Yates W R, Troughton E, *et al* (1995) **Genetic-environmental interaction in the genesis of aggressivity and conduct disorders**. *Archives of General Psychiatry*, **52**, 916–924.

Dodge K A , J E Bates, Pettit G S, *et al* (1990) **Mechanisms in the cycle of violence**. *Science*, **250**, 1678–1683.

Farrington D P (1995) **The development of offending and antisocial behaviour from childhood: key findings from the Cambridge study in delinquent development**. *Journal of Child Psychology and Psychiatry*, **36**, 929–964.

Holland R, Moretti M M, Verlaan V, *et al* (1993) **Attachment and conduct disorder: the Response Program**. *Canadian Journal of Psychiatry*, **38**, 420–431.

Loeber R (1991) **Antisocial behaviour: more enduring than changeable?** *Journal of the American Academy of Child and Adolescent Psychiatry*, **30**, 393–397.

——, Green S M, Keenan K, *et al* (1995) **Which boys will fare worse? Early predictors of the onset of conduct disorder in a six-year longitudinal study**. *Journal of the American Academy of Child and Adolescent Psychiatry*, **34**, 499–509.

Lyons-Ruth K (1996) **Attachment relationships among children with aggressive behavior problems: The role of disorganized early attachment patterns**. *Journal of Consulting and Clinical Psychology*, **64**, 64–73.

Lytton H (1990) **Child and parent effects in boys' conduct disorder: A reinterpretation**. *Developmental-Psychology*, **26**, 683–697.

McCord J (1978) **A thirty-year follow up of treatment effects**. *American Psychologist*, **33**, 284–289.

Moffitt T E (1993) **Adolescence-limited and life-course-persistent antisocial behavior: A developmental taxonomy**. *Psychological Review*, **100**, 674–701.

Patterson G R (1982) *Coercive Family Process*. Eugene, OR: Castalia.

——, Chamberlain P A & Reid J B (1982) **A comparative evaluation of a parent-training program**. *Behavior Therapy*, **13**, 638–650.

Quinton D, Pickles A, Maughan B, *et al* (1993) **Partners, peers, and pathways: Assortative pairing and continuities in conduct disorder**. *Development and Psychopathology*, **5**, 763–783.

Raine A, Brennan P, Mednick S A, *et al* (1994) **Birth complications combined with early maternal rejection at age 1 year predispose to violent crime at age 18 years**. *Archives of General Psychiatry*, **51**, 984–988.

Robins L N (1978) **Sturdy childhood predictors of adult antisocial behavior: replications from the longitudinal studies**. *Psychological Medicine*, **8**, 611–622.

Routh C P, Hill J W, Steele H, *et al* (1995) **Maternal attachment status, psychosocial stressors and problem behaviour: Follow-up after parent training courses for conduct disorder**. *Journal of Child Psychology and Psychiatry and Allied Disciplines*, **36**, 1179–1198.

Rutter M (1990) **Psychosocial resilience and protective mechanisms**. In *Risk and Protective Factors in the Development of Psychopathology* (eds J Rolf, A S Masten, D Cicchetti *et al*), pp. 181–214. New York: Cambridge University Press.

Silberg J L, Rutter, M, Meyer J, *et al* (1996) **Genetic and environmental influences on the covariation between hyperactivity and conduct disturbance in juvenile twins**. *Journal of Child Psychology and Psychiatry and Allied Disciplines*, **37**, 803–816.

Taylor E, Chadwick O, Heptinstall E, *et al* (1996) **Hyperactivity and conduct problems as risk factors for adolescent development**. *Journal of the American Academy of Child and Adolescent Psychiatry*, **35**, 1213–1226.

van den Boom D C (1995) **Do first-year intervention effects endure? Follow-up during toddlerhood of a sample of Dutch irritable infants**. *Child Development*, **66**, 1798–1816.

Webster-Stratton C (1997) **Treating children with early-onset conduct problems: a comparison of child and parent training interventions**. *Journal of Consulting and Clinical Psychology*, **65**, 93–109.

——, Hollingsworth T & Kolpacoff M (1989) **The long-term effectiveness and clinical significance of three cost-effective training programs for families with conduct-problem children**. *Journal of Consulting and Clinical Psychology*, **57**, 550–553.

Zoccolillo M, Pickles A, Quinton D, *et al* (1992) **The outcome of childhood conduct disorder: Implications for defining adult personality disorder and conduct disorder**. *Psychological Medicine*, **22**, 971–986.

● CUTTING EDGE PAPERS ●

Belsky J, Hsieh K H, Crnic K, *et al* (1998) **Mothering, fathering, and infant negativity as antecedents of boys' externalizing problems and inhibition at age 3 years: Differential susceptibility to rearing experience?** *Development and Psychopathology*, **10**, 301–319.

Bennett K J, Lipman E L, Brown S, *et al* (1999) **Predicting conduct problems: Can high-risk children be identified in kindergarten and Grade 1?** *Journal of Consulting and Clinical Psychology*, **67**, 470–480.

Boyle M H & Willms J D (2001) **Multilevel modelling of hierarchical data in developmental studies**. *Journal of Child Psychology and Psychiatry and Allied Disciplines*, **42**, 141–162.

Campbell S B, Shaw D S & Gilliom M (2000) **Early externalizing behavior problems: Toddlers and preschoolers at risk for later maladjustment**. *Development and Psychopathology*, **12**, 467–488.

Chamberlain P & Moore K (1998) **A clinical model for parenting juvenile offenders: A comparison of group care versus family care**. *Clinical Child Psychology and Psychiatry*, **3**, 375–386.

Conduct Problems Prevention Research Group (1999) **Initial impact of the fast track prevention trial for conduct problems: I. The high-risk sample**. *Journal of Consulting and Clinical Psychology*, **67**, 631–647.

Dishion T J, McCord J, Poulin F, *et al* (1999) **When interventions harm: Peer groups and problem behavior**. *American Psychologist*, **54**, 755–764.

Farrington D P (1999) **A criminological research agenda for the next millennium**. *International Journal of Offender Therapy and Comparative Criminology*, **43**, 154–167.

Fergusson D M & Horwood L J (1998) **Early conduct problems and later life opportunities**. *Journal of Child Psychology and Psychiatry and Allied Disciplines*, **39**, 1097–1108.

Fergusson D M & Lynskey M T (1998) **Conduct problems in childhood and psychosocial outcomes in young adulthood: A prospective study**. *Journal of Emotional and Behavioral Disorders*, **6**, 2–18.

——, Woodward L J, Horwood L J, *et al* (1998) **Maternal smoking during pregnancy and psychiatric adjustment in late adolescence**. *Archives of General Psychiatry*, **55**, 721–727.

Findling R L, McNamara N K, Branicky L A, *et al* (2000) **A double-blind pilot study of risperidone in the treatment of conduct disorder**. *Journal of the American Academy of Child and Adolescent Psychiatry*, **39**, 509–516.

Gardner F, Sonuga-Barke E & Sayal K (1999) **Parents anticipating misbehavior: An observational study of strategies parents use to prevent conflict with behavior problem children**. *Journal of Child Psychology and Psychiatry*, **40**, 1185–1196.

Harrington R, Peters S, Green J, *et al* (2000) **Randomised comparison of the effectiveness and costs of community and hospital based mental health services for children with behavioural disorders**. *British Medical Journal*, **321**, 1047–1050.

Huesmann L R, Maxwell C D, Eron L, *et al* (1996) **Evaluating a cognitive/ ecological program for the prevention of aggression among urban children**. *American Journal of Preventive Medicine*, **12** (suppl.), 120–128.

Huey S J, Henggeler S W, Brondino M J, *et al* (2000) **Mechanisms of change in multisystemic therapy: Reducing delinquent behavior through therapist adherence and improved family and peer functioning**. *Journal of Consulting and Clinical Psychology*, **68**, 451–467.

Hughes C & Dunn J (2000) **Hedonism or empathy? Hard-to-manage children's moral awareness and links with cognitive and maternal characteristics**. *British Journal of Developmental Psychology*, **18**, 227–245.

——, ——, White A J, *et al* (1998) **Trick or treat? Uneven understanding of mind and emotion and executive dysfunction in hard-to-manage preschoolers**. *Journal of Child Psychology and Psychiatry and Allied Disciplines*, **39**, 981–994.

——, White A, Sharpen J, *et al* (2000) **Antisocial, angry and unsympathetic: Hard to manage preschoolers' peer problems and possible cognitive influences**. *Journal of Child Psychology and Psychiatry and Allied Disciplines*, **41**, 169–179.

Kazdin A E & Wassell G (1999) **Barriers to treatment participation and therapeutic change among children referred for conduct disorder**. *Journal of Clinical Child Psychology*, **28**, 160–172.

Lahey B B, Waldman I D & McBurnett K (1999) **Annotation: the development of antisocial behaviour: An integrative causal model**. *Journal of Child Psychology and Psychiatry*, **40**, 669–682.

Loeber R, Green S M, Lahey B B, *et al* (2000) **Findings on disruptive behavior disorders from the first decade of the Developmental Trends Study**. *Clinical Child and Family Psychology Review*, **3**, 37–60.

Malone R P, Delaney M A, Leubbert J F, *et al* (2000) **A double-blind placebo-controlled study of lithium in hospitalized aggressive children and adolescents with conduct disorder**. *Archives of General Psychiatry*, **57**, 649–654.

McBurnett, K, Lahey B B, Capasso L, *et al* (2000) **Low salivary cortisol and persistent aggression in boys referred for disruptive behavior**. *Archives of General Psychiatry*, **57**, 38–43.

Murray L, Sinclair D, Cooper P, *et al* (1999) **The socioemotional development of 5 year old children of postnatally depressed mothers**. *Journal of Child Psychology and Psychiatry and Allied Disciplines*, **40**, 1259–1271.

Nix R L, Pinderhughes E E, Dodge K A, *et al* (1999) **The relation between mothers' hostile attribution tendencies and children's externalizing behavior problems: The mediating role of mothers' harsh discipline practices**. *Child Development*, **70**, 896–909.

Pettit G S, Bates J E, Dodge K A, *et al* (1997) **Supportive parenting, ecological context, and children's adjustment: A seven-year longitudinal study**. *Child Development*, **68**, 908–923.

Rutter M L (1999) **Psychosocial adversity and child psychopathology**. *British Journal of Psychiatry*, **174**, 480–493.

Sanders M R, Markie-Dadds C, Tully L A, *et al* (2000) **The Triple P – Positive Parenting Program: A comparison of enhanced, standard, and self-directed behavioral family intervention for parents of children with early onset conduct problems**. *Journal of Consulting and Clinical Psychology*, **68**, 624–640.

Shaw D S, Winslow E B, Owens E B, *et al* (1998) **The development of early externalizing problems among children from low-income families: A transformational perspective**. *Journal of Abnormal Child Psychology*, **26**, 95–107.

Stoolmiller M, Eddy J M, Reid J B, *et al* (2000) **Detecting and describing preventive intervention effects in a universal school-based randomized trial targeting delinquent and violent behavior**. *Journal of Consulting and Clinical Psychology*, **68**, 296–306.

Street C (2000) *Whose Crisis? Meeting the Needs of Children and Young People with Serious Mental Health Problems*. London: Young Minds.

Taylor T K , Schmidt F, Pepler D, *et al* (1998) A **comparison of eclectic treatment with Webster-Stratton's parents and children series in a children's mental health center: A randomized controlled trial**. *Behavior Therapy*, **29**, 221–240.

● BOOKS ●

Farrington D P (1999) **Conduct disorder and delinquency**. In *Risks and outcomes in Developmental Psychopathology* (eds H C Steinhausen & F C Verhulst), pp. 165–192. Oxford: Oxford University Press.

—— & Loeber R (1999) **Transatlantic replicability of risk factors in the development of delinquency**. In *Historical and Geographical Influences on Psychopathology* (ed. P Cohen), pp. 299–329. Mahwah, NJ: Lawrence Erlbaum Associates.

Kazdin A (1985) *Treatment of Antisocial Behaviour in Children and Adolescents*. Homewood, IL: Dorsey.

Loeber R & Farrington D P (1998) *Serious and Violent Juvenile Offenders: Risk Factors and Successful Interventions*. Thousand Oaks, CA: Sage Publications.

Robins L N (1999) **A 70-year history of conduct disorder: Variations in definitions, prevalence, and correlates**. In *Historical and Geographical Influences on Psychopathology* (ed. P Cohen), pp. 37–56. Mahwah, NJ: Lawrence Erlbaum Associates.

Rutter M, Giller H, Hagell A, *et al* (1998) *Antisocial Behavior by Young People*. New York: Cambridge University Press.

Werner E E & Smith R S (1992) *Overcoming the Odds: High Risk Children from Birth to Adulthood*. Ithaca, NY: Cornell University Press.

Cochrane Controlled Trials Register
109 hits (keywords: "conduct disorder")
153 hits (key words: "conduct disorder*")
45 hits (key words: "aggressive behaviour")
252 hits (key words: "aggressive behavior")
100 hits (key words: "aggressive behavior" AND child*)

Cochrane Developmental, Psychosocial and Learning Problems Group
Contact: Dr Jane Dennis, Bristol, UK. J.Dennis@bristol.ac.uk

DELIBERATE SELF-HARM

INTRODUCTION

Deliberate self-harm involves any intentional act to cause harm to oneself. The main forms of deliberate self-harm are self-injury and self-poisoning. Self-harm can include overdoses of drugs or alcohol, pulling hair, cutting or picking of the skin and self-strangulation. The most common form of deliberate self-harm is self-poisoning.[46]

Deliberate self-harm or suicide is more common in girls than in boys between the ages of 10 and 14 years.[47]

AETIOLOGY

Children most at risk are those who have disturbed family relationships (especially alcohol misuse). Often, personality and psychiatric problems increase the likelihood of self-harm. Specific stressful events can also precipitate the incidence of self-harm.[48]

REFERENCES

● SYSTEMATIC REVIEWS AND META-ANALYSES ●

Chance S E, Kaslow N J, Summerville M B, *et al* (1998) **Suicidal behavior in African American individuals: current status and future directions**. *Cultural Diversity in Mental Health*, **4**, 19–37.

Hawton K, Arensman E, Townsend E, *et al* (1998) **Deliberate self harm: systematic review of efficacy of psychosocial and pharmacological treatments in preventing repetition**. *British Medical Journal*, **317**, 441–447.

——, Townsend,E, Arensman E, *et al* (2000) **Psychosocial and pharmacological treatments for deliberate self harm**. Cochrane Review. In *The Cochrane Library*, Issue 4. Oxford: Update Software.

Ploeg J, Ciliska D, Dobbins M, *et al* (1996) **A systematic overview of adolescent suicide prevention programs**. *Canadian Journal of Public Health*, **87**, 319–324.

Van der Sande R, Buskens E, Allart E, *et al* (1997) **Psychosocial intervention following suicide attempt: A systematic review of treatment interventions**. *Acta Psychiatrica Scandinavica*, **96**, 43–50.

● REVIEWS ●

Shaffer D & Piacentini J (1994) **Suicide and attempted suicide**. In *Child and Adolescent Psychiatry: Modern Approaches* (eds M Rutter, E Taylor & L Hersov), pp. 407–424. Oxford: Blackwell Scientific Publications.

---

46   NHS Centre for Reviews and Dissemination (1998) Deliberate self-harm. *Effective Health Care,* **4**.

47   Hawton K *et al* (1982) cited in Black D, Cottrell D, Kaplan T, *et al* (1993) Liaison child and adolescent psychiatry. In *Seminars in Child and Adolescent Psychiatry* (eds D Black & D Cottrell), pp. 249–275. London: Gaskell.

48   Scarth L (1993) Clinical syndromes in adolescence. In *Seminars in Child and Adolescent Psychiatry* (eds D Black & D Cottrell), pp. 154–182. London: Gaskell.

● CLASSIC PAPERS ●

Centers for Disease Control (1991) **Attempted suicide among high school students – United States**. *Morbidity and Mortality Weekly Report*, **4**, 633–635.

Shaffer D (1974) **Suicide in childhood and early adolescence**. *Journal of Child Psychology and Psychiatry*, **15**, 275–291.

—, Gould M, Fisher P, *et al* (1996) **Psychiatric diagnosis in child and adolescent suicide**. *Archives of General Psychiatry*, **53**, 339–348.

● REPORTS ●

NHS Health Advisory Service (1994) ***Suicide Prevention – The Challenge Confronted***. London: HMSO.

Royal College of Psychiatrists (1994) ***Consensus Guidelines on the General Hospital Management of Deliberate Self-Harm Patients***. London: The Royal College of Psychiatrists.

Royal College of Psychiatrists (1998) ***Managing Deliberate Self-harm in Young People***. Council Report CR64. London: The Royal College of Psychiatrists.

Schmidtke A, Bille-Brahe U, Deleo D, *et al* (1996) **Attempted suicide in Europe: rates, trends, and socio-demographic characteristics of suicide attempters during the period 1989–1992. Results of the WHO/EURO Multicentre Study on Parasuicide**. *Acta Psychiatrica Scandinavica*, **93**, 327–338.

● NEW RESEARCH AND THEORIES ●

Dicker R, Morrisey R F, Abikoff H, *et al* (1997) **Hospitalizing the suicidal adolescent: decision-making criteria of psychiatric residents**. *Journal of the American Academy of Child and Adolescent Psychiatry*, **36**, 769–776.

Fombonne E (1998) **Suicidal behaviour in vulnerable adolescents. Time trends and their correlates**. *British Journal of Psychiatry*, **173**, 154–159.

Harrington R, Kerfoot M, Dyer E, *et al* (1998) **Randomised trial of family intervention for children who have deliberately poisoned themselves**. *Journal of the American Academy of Child and Adolescent Psychiatry*, **37**, 512–518.

Negron R, Placentini J, Graae F, *et al* (1997) **Microanalysis of adolescent suicide attempters and ideators during the acute suicide episode**. *Journal of the American Academy of Child and Adolescent Psychiatry*, **36**, 1512–1519.

Peterson B S, Zhang H, Santa Lucia R, *et al* (1996) **Risk factors for presenting problems in child psychiatric emergencies**. *Journal of the American Academy of Child and Adolescent Psychiatry*, **35**, 1162–1173.

Shaffer D, Gould M S, Fisher P, *et al* (1996) **Psychiatric diagnosis in child and adolescent suicide**. *Archives of General Psychiatry*, **53**, 339–348.

Stein D, Apter A, Ratzoni G, *et al* (1998) **Association between multiple suicide attempts and negative affects in adolescents**. *Journal of the American Academy of Child and Adolescent Psychiatry*, **37**, 488–494.

● USEFUL WEBSITES ●

Suicide Awareness/Voice of Education (SAVE) http://www.save.org

Cochrane Controlled Trials Register
8 hits (keywords: "self harm" AND child*)
15 hits (keywords: "self harm" AND adolesc*)
31 hits (keywords: suicid* AND child*)

Cochrane Depression, Anxiety and Neurosis Group
Contact: Dr Natalie Khin, Review Group Coordinator, New Zealand.
n.khin@auckland.ac.nz

EATING DISORDERS

INTRODUCTION

Eating disorders are characterised by obsession with size, distorted body image, high levels of activity, preoccupation with food and the failure to acknowledge an eating problem.[49] Eating disorders are also associated with depressive symptoms, social withdrawal, insomnia, irritability and obsessive–compulsive features, as well as features of personality disorders. The onset of an eating disorder is typically between the ages of 14 and 18 years. The two main forms of eating disorders are anorexia nervosa and bulimia nervosa.

Anorexia nervosa is characterised by the inability to maintain a healthy body weight. **Bulimia nervosa** is associated with normal weight or being slightly under or overweight and involves episodes of binge eating followed by compensatory behaviours such as self-induced vomiting, abuse of laxatives or diuretics and excessive exercise.

Anorexia nervosa is reported to occur in 0.2–1.0% of the 12–19-year-old population, and is 8–11 times more common in females than males.[50] Bulimia nervosa is more common than anorexia nervosa and occurs in approximately 2.5% of the population of girls and boys between the ages of 13 and 18 years. It is far more common in girls than boys.[51] In a recent survey of children in Great Britain by the Office of National Statistics, it was estimated that eating disorders occur in 1% of the population of children and adolescents.[52]

DIAGNOSIS AND AETIOLOGY

The ICD–10 criteria for diagnosis of anorexia must include:

○ a body mass index of 17.5 or lower;

○ self-induced weight loss through the avoidance of certain foods, self-induced vomiting or purging, excessive exercise, use of appetite suppressants and/or diuretics;

○ distortion of body image;

○ amenorrhoea in women or a loss of sexual interest and potency in men; and

○ delayed growth if onset is before puberty.

The DSM–IV–TR categories are similar to the ICD–10 categories but include two categories of anorexia nervosa that are of either the restricting type or binge-eating/purging type.

49 Scarth L (1993) **Clinical syndromes in adolescence**. In *Seminars in Child and Adolescent Psychiatry* (eds D Black & D Cottrell), 154–182. London: Gaskell.

50 Nielson S (1990) cited in Wallace W A, Crown J M, Berger M, *et al* (1997) **Child and adolescent mental health: Health care needs assessment**. In *The Epidemiologically Based Needs Assessment Reviews* (eds A Stevens & J Raftery). 2nd series. Oxon: Radcliffe Medical Press.

51 Steinhausen *et al* (1992) cited in Wallace W A, Crown J M, Berger M, *et al* (1997) **Child and adolescent mental health: Health care needs assessment**. In *The Epidemiologically Based Needs Assessment Reviews* (eds A Stevens & J Raftery). 2nd series. Oxon: Radcliffe Medical Press.

52 Meltzer H, Gatward R, Goodman R, *et al* (2000) *The Mental Health of Children and Adolescents in Great Britain*. London: The Stationery Office.

Criteria for diagnosis of bulimia nervosa according to the ICD–10 include:

○ preoccupation with eating and an irresistible craving for food with episodes of overeating;

○ self-induced vomiting; purgative abuse, alternating periods of starvation, use of appetite suppressants, thyroid preparations or diuretics; and

○ distortion of body image.

The aetiology of eating disorders can include individual, familial, sociocultural and biological factors as well as precipitating events and perpetuating factors.

CRITICAL QUESTIONS

by Professor Bryan Lask

What developments have there been in the management of eating disorders in the past 2–5 years?

The complexity and severity of early-onset eating disorders continue to present a major challenge to children's health and to carers, clinicians and researchers. Family-based treatments remain central to any management programme. Evidence is emerging of primary abnormalities in cerebral functioning as well as the secondary changes owing to starvation and dehydration. The significance of the primary changes has yet to be ascertained. Primary prevention programmes focused on eating behaviour in adolescents have no value and may even lead to an increase in dietary restraint.

What are the key messages from new research that are not being widely used?

○ Treatment should be focused on the family as much as on the individual.

○ Motivational interviewing and motivational enhancement theories are likely to play an increasingly important part in the management of eating disorders, and every effort should be made to adjust programmes to the individual's level of motivation and insight.

○ Further understanding is required of the neurobiological changes noted on brain imaging.

REFERENCES

● CLINICAL EVIDENCE ●

Anorexia nervosa has been commissioned for a future edition.

Hay P & Bacaltchuk J (2000) **Bulimia nervosa**. In *Clinical evidence: A Compendium of the Best Available Evidence for Effective Health Care*. Issue 4, pp. 511–518. London: BMJ Publishing Group.

● SYSTEMATIC REVIEWS AND META-ANALYSES ●

Allison D B & Faith M S (1996) **Hypnosis as an adjunct to cognitive behavioural psychotherapy: a meta-analytic reappraisal**. *Journal of Consulting and Clinical Psychology*, **64**, 513–516. (Reviewed on DARE.)

Campbell K, Summerbell C, O'Meara S, *et al* (1999) **Interventions for treating obesity in children**. Cochrane Review. In *The Cochrane Library*, Issue 4. Oxford: Update Software.

——, Waters E, O'Meara S, *et al* (1999) **Interventions for preventing obesity in children**. Cochrane Review Update. In *The Cochrane Library*, Issue 4. Oxford: Update Software.

Epstein L H, Cloeman K J & Myers M D (1996) **Exercise in treating obesity in children and adolescents**. *Medicine and Science in Sports and Exercise*, **28**, 428–435. (Reviewed on DARE.)

Fombonne E (1995) **Anorexia nervosa: no evidence of an increase**. *British Journal of Psychiatry*, **166**, 462–471.

Glenny A M (1997) **The treatment of obesity: A systematic review of the literature**. *International Journal of Obesity Related Metabolic Disorders*, **21**, 715–737.

—— & O'Meara S (1997) **Systematic review of interventions in the treatment and prevention of obesity**. *CRD Report*, **10**, 1–149. (Reviewed on DARE.)

——, Melville A, O'Meara S, *et al* (1997) **The treatment and prevention of obesity: a systematic review of the literature**. *International Journal of Obesity and Related Metabolic Disorders*, **21**, 715–737.

Harvey E L, Glenny A, Kirk S F L, *et al* (1999) **Improving health professionals' management and the organization of care for overweight people**. Cochrane Review. In *The Cochrane Library*, Issue 1. Oxford: Update Software.

Hay P & Bacaltchuk J (2001) **Psychotherapy for bulimia nervosa and binging**. Cochrane Review. In *The Cochrane Library*, Issue 1. Oxford: Update Software.

Jacobi C (1997) **Comparison of controlled psycho- and pharmacotherapy studies in bulimia and anorexia nervosa**. *Psychotherapy and Psychosomatic Medicine in Psychology*, **47**, 346–364.

Kirsh I (1996) **Hypnotic enhancement of cognitive–behavioural weight loss treatments – another meta-reanalysis**. *Journal of Consulting and Clinical Psychology*, **64**, 517–519.

——, Montgomery G & Sapirstein G (1995) **Hypnosis as an adjunct to cognitive–behavioural psychotherapy: a meta-analysis**. *Journal of Consulting and Clinical Psychology*, **63**, 214–220. (Reviewed on DARE.)

Lewandowski L M (1997) **Meta-analysis of cognitive–behavioral treatment studies for bulimia**. *Clinical Psychology Review*, **17**, 703–718.

Murnen S K & Smolak L (1997) **Femininity, masculinity, and disordered eating: a meta-analytic review**. *International Journal of Eating Disorders*, **22**, 231–242.

Parsons T J, Power C, Logan S, *et al* (1999) **Childhood predictors of adult obesity: a systematic review**. *International Journal of Obesity and Related Metabolic Disorders*, **23** (suppl. 8), S1–107.

Schoemaker C (1997) **Does early intervention improve the prognosis in anorexia nervosa? A systematic review of the treatment-outcome literature**. *International Journal of Eating Disorders*, **21**, 1–15. (Reviewed on DARE.)

Smolak L, Murnen S K & Ruble A E (2000) **Female athletes and eating problems: a meta-analysis**. *International Journal of Eating Disorders*, **27**, 371–380.

Summerbell C D, Waters E, O'Meara S, *et al* (2001) **Interventions for treating obesity in children**. Cochrane Review. In *The Cochrane Library*, Issue 2. Oxford: Update Software.

Wonderlich S A, Brewerton T D, Jocic J, *et al* (1997) **Relationship of childhood sexual abuse and eating disorders**. *Journal of the American Academy of Child and Adolescent Psychiatry*, **36**, 1107–1115.

● PRACTICE PARAMETERS ●

American Psychiatric Association (1993) **Practice guidelines for eating disorders**. *American Journal of Psychiatry*, **150**, 207–228.

● REVIEWS ●

Lask B & Bryant-Waugh R (1995) **Eating disorders in children**. *Journal of Child Psychology and Psychiatry*, **36**, 191–202.

Steiner H & Lock J (1998) **Anorexia nervosa and bulimia nervosa in children and adolescents: a review of the past 10 years**. *Journal of the American Academy of Child and Adolescent Psychiatry*, **37**, 352–359.

Steinhausen H C (1997) **Annotation: Outcome of anorexia nervosa in the younger patient**. *Journal of Child Psychology and Psychiatry*, **38**, 271–276.

● CLASSIC PAPERS ●

Katzman D & Zipursky R (1997) **Adolescents with anorexia nervosa: the impact of the disorder on bones and brains. Adolescent nutritional disorders prevention and treatment**. *Annals of the New York Academy of Sciences*, **817**, 127–133.

Russell G (1985) **Premenarchal anorexia nervosa and its sequelae**. *Journal of Psychiatric Research*, **19**, 363–369.

——, Smzukler G I, Dare C, *et al* (1987) **An evaluation of family therapy in anorexia nervosa and bulimia nervosa**. *Archives of General Psychiatry*, **44**, 1047–1056.

● CUTTING EDGE PAPERS ●

Eisler I, Dare C, Russell G F, *et al* (1997) **Family and individual therapy in anorexia nervosa: a five year follow-up**. *Archives of General Psychiatry*, **54**, 1025–1030.

Gordon I, Lask B, Bryant-Waugh R, *et al* (1997) **Anorexia nervosa in children: evidence of primary limbic abnormality**. *International Journal of Eating Disorders*, **22**, 159–165.

Nicholls D, Chater R & Lask B (2000) **Children into DSM don't do: A comparison of classification systems of eating disorders for children**. *International Journal of Eating Disorders*, **28**, 317–324.

Strober M, Freeman R & Morrell W (1997) **The long term course of severe anorexia nervosa in adolescents: Survival analysis of recovery, relapse and outcome predicted over 10–15 years in a prospective study**. *International Journal of Eating Disorders*, **22**, 339–360.

● REPORTS ●

NHS Centre for Reviews and Dissemination (1997) **The prevention and treatment of obesity**. *Effective Health Care*, **3**, 1–12.

Office of Health Economics (1994) *Eating Disorders*. London: Office of Health Economics.

● BOOKS ●

Bryant-Waugh R & Lask B (1999) *Eating Disorders: A Parent's Guide*. London: Penguin. (Also published in Italian.)

Lask B & Bryant-Waugh R (eds) (2000) *Anorexia Nervosa and Related Eating Disorders in Childhood and Adolescence*. 2nd edn. Hove, UK: Psychology Press.

● FOCUS REPORT ●

Fox C & Joughin C (in press) *Childhood-Onset Eating Problems: Findings from the Evidence*. London: Gaskell.

● USEFUL WEBSITES ●

Eating Disorders Association http://gurney.co.uk/eda/

Eating Disorders Shared Awareness (EDSA) http://eating-disorder.com

---

Cochrane Controlled Trials Register
64 hits (keywords: "eating disorder*" AND child)
120 hits (keywords: "eating disorder*" AND adolesc*)
64 hits (keywords: bulimia OR "anorexia nervosa" AND adolesc*)

ELIMINATION

INTRODUCTION

There are two types of disorders that fall under the heading 'elimination'. These are (1) enuresis and (2) faecal soiling.

Enuresis is the repeated and involuntary passing of urine during sleep in children over five years of age who do not have any physical abnormality. Enuresis can be nocturnal, diurnal or a combination of both.

Faecal soiling refers to disorders of the bowl function and control that are not a result of any physical abnormality or disease.[53] Faecal soiling usually applies to children over the age of four years, but the age at which bowl control is obtained varies across cultures. Behaviours can include lack of bowl control and/or the inappropriate placement of faeces once control is obtained. The word 'encopresis' is often used to describe the various behaviours associated with faecal soiling.

Nocturnal enuresis occurs in approximately 15–20% of five-year-olds, 7% of seven-year-olds, 5% of 10-year-olds and 2–3% of 12–14-year-olds. Only 1–2% of children aged 15 years or over will occasionally suffer from nocturnal enuresis.[54]

Faecal soiling is more common in boys than girls[55]. It is estimated that encopresis occurs in approximately 4.7% of children and 0.7% of adolescents in England.[56]

DIAGNOSIS AND AETIOLOGY

The aetiology of enuresis is associated with various factors. These include genetic influences, circadian rhythms, bladder size and function, developmental changes or delays, sleep abnormalities, toilet training or stressful experiences. There also appears to be some evidence of a neuropharmacological basis of enuresis.

For the diagnosis of enuresis according to the DSM–IV–TR, a child must be five years of age or older and repeatedly pass urine at any time of the day into his or her bed or clothes at least twice a week for at least three months. The symptoms should not be accounted for by medication or a medical condition and must cause significant distress in areas of functioning.

For the diagnosis of encopresis (faecal soiling) according to the DSM–IV–TR, a child must be four years of age or older and repeatedly pass faeces in inappropriate places at least once a month for three months.

Unlike the DSM–IV–TR, the ICD–10 does not have a separate category for elimination disorders but has a category called 'Other behavioural and emotional disorders with onset usually occurring in childhood or adolescence' and includes categories for nonorganic enuresis and nonorganic encopresis similar to those in the DSM–IV–TR.

---

53 Hersov L (1994) Faecal soiling. In *Child and Adolescent Psychiatry: Modern Approaches* (eds M Rutter, E Taylor & L Hersov). 3rd edn. Oxford: Blackwell Scientific Publications.

54 Blackwell C (1989) cited in Bosson S & Lynth N (2000) Nocturnal enuresis. In *Clinical Evidence: A Compendium of the Best Available Evidence for Effective Health Care*. Issue 3. London: BMJ Publishing Group.

55 Berelowitz M & Nelki J (1993) Clinical syndromes in middle childhood. In *Seminars in Child and Adolescent Psychiatry* (eds D Black & D Cottrell), pp. 124–153. London: Gaskell.

56 Kurtz Z, Thornes R & Wolkind S (1996) *Services for the Mental Health of Children and Young People in England: A National Review*. Report to the Department of Health. London: South West Thames Regional Health Authority.

The aetiology of faecal soiling can include premature toilet training and developmental delays, as well as family conflict. Sexual abuse should be also be considered as a possible cause of the disorder.

REFERENCES

● CLINICAL EVIDENCE ●

Bosson S & Lynth N (2000) **Nocturnal enuresis**. In *Clinical Evidence: A Compendium of the Best Available Evidence for Effective Health Care*, Issue 4, pp. 231–235. London: BMJ Publishing Group.

Rubin G (2000) **Constipation in children**. In *Clinical Evidence: A Compendium of the Best Available Evidence for Effective Health Care*, Issue 4, pp. 201–205. London: BMJ Publishing Group.

● SYSTEMATIC REVIEWS AND META-ANALYSES ●

Brazzelli M & Griffith P (2000) **Behavioural and cognitive interventions for faecal incontinence in children**. Protocol for Cochrane Review. In *The Cochrane Library*, Issue 4. Oxford: Update Software.

Glazener C M & Evans J H (2000) **Tricyclic and related drugs for nocturnal enuresis in children**. Cochrane Review. In *The Cochrane Library*, Issue 4. Oxford: Update Software.

—— & —— (2000) **Desmopressin for nocturnal enuresis in children**. Cochrane Review. In *The Cochrane Library*, Issue 4. Oxford: Update Software.

—— & —— (2000) **Drugs for nocturnal enuresis in children (other than desmopressin and tricyclics)**. Cochrane Review. In *The Cochrane Library*, Issue 4. Oxford: Update Software.

Lister-Sharp D, O'Meara S, Bradley M, *et al* (1997) **A systematic review of the effectiveness of interventions for managing childhood nocturnal enuresis**. *CRD*, Report 11. York: NHS Centre for Reviews and Dissemination, University of York.

Price K (2000) **What is the role of stimulant laxatives in the management of childhood constipation and soiling?** Protocol for Cochrane Review. In *The Cochrane Library*, Issue 4. Oxford: Update Software.

Sureshkumar P, Bower W, Craig J C, *et al* (2000) **Treatment of daytime urinary incontinence in children**. Protocol for Cochrane Review. In *The Cochrane Library*, Issue 4. Oxford: Update Software.

● CLINICAL GUIDELINES ●

Felt B, Wise C G, Olson A, *et al* (1999) **Guideline for the management of paediatric idiopathic constipation and soiling**. *Archives of Paediatric and Adolescent Medicine*, **153**, 380–385.

● REVIEWS ●

Butler R J (1998) **Annotation: Night wetting in children: Psychological aspects**. *Journal of Child Psychology and Psychiatry*, **39**, 453–463.

Clayden G S (1992) **Management of chronic constipation**. *Archives of Disease in Childhood*, **67**, 340–344.

Kelly C P (1996) **Chronic constipation and soiling: a review of the psychological and family literature**. *Child Psychology and Psychiatry Review*, 1, 59–66.

Levine M D, & Backow H (1976) **Children with encopresis: a study of treatment outcome**. *Pediatrics*, **58**, 845–897.

von Gontard A (1998) **Day and night wetting in children – a paediatric and child psychiatry perspective**. *Journal of Child Psychology and Psychiatry*, **39**, 439–451.

● CLASSIC PAPERS ●

Anthony E J (1957) **An experimental approach to the psychopathology of childhood: encopresis**. *British Journal of Medical Psychology*, **30**, 146–175.

Berg I, Forsyth I, Holt P, *et al* (1982) **A controlled trial of 'Senokot' in faecal soiling treated with behavioural methods**. *Journal of Child Psychology and Psychiatry*, **149**, 543–549.

Levine M D (1975) **Children with encopresis: a descriptive analysis**. *Pediatrics*, **56**, 412–416.

White M (1984) **Pseudo-encopresis: from avalanche to victory, from vicious to virtuous cycles**. *Family Systems Medicine*, **2**, 150–160.

● CUTTING EDGE PAPERS ●

Cox D J, Borowitz S, Kovatchev B, *et al* (1998) **Contributions of behaviour therapy and biofeedback to laxative therapy in the treatment of paediatric encopresis**. *Annals of Behavioural Medicine*, **20**, 70–76.

Stark L J, Opipari L C, Donaldson D L, *et al* (1997) **Evaluation of a standard protocol for retentive encopresis: a replication**. *Journal of Pediatric Psychology*, **22**, 619–633.

Cochrane Controlled Trials Register
25 hits (keywords: encopresis AND child*)
259 hits (keywords: enuresis AND child*)

Cochrane Developmental, Psychosocial and Learning Problems Group
Contact: Dr Jane Dennis, Bristol, UK. J.Dennis@bristol.ac.uk

INTRODUCTION

Anxiety has a different mode of presentation in children than in adults and symptoms are dependent on the developmental level of the child. At an early age, anxiety may arise from being separated from caregivers. In the later years, anxiety can include being frightened of particular situations, such as the dark, and may cause physical complaints such as stomach aches or headaches. Anxiety may also cause children to engage in behaviours associated with an earlier developmental stage.

Separation anxiety disorder occurs in approximately 0.9% of boys and 0.7% of girls and generalized anxiety disorder in 0.5% of boys and 0.7% of girls in Great Britain according to a recent survey by the Office of National Statistics.[57]

Phobias are conditions where there is an inappropriate fear of specific objects or situations[58]. Simple phobias are estimated to occur in 2.3%–9.2% of children.[59] Specific phobias occur in 0.9% of boys and 1.1% of girls, social phobias in 0.4% of boys and 0.3% of girls and agoraphobia in 0.1% of all children in Great Britain.[60]

DIAGNOSIS AND AETIOLOGY

The ICD–10 identifies four main types of anxiety disorders in childhood. These are: separation anxiety; phobic anxiety; social anxiety; and sibling rivalry.[61] The DSM–IV–TR only has one category for anxiety disorders in infancy, childhood or adolescence which is separation anxiety disorder. Childhood and adolescence occurrence of phobias are included in the adult category of social phobias[62] and sibling relational problems fall under the category of 'Relational problems'.[63]

CRITICAL QUESTIONS

by Dr Ian Wilkinson

What developments have there been in the management of anxiety and phobia in the past 2–5 years?

The most useful developments are not so much to do with new theories but the application of existing knowledge to preventive psychoeducational strategies via families and in the classroom.

57   Meltzer H, Gatward R, Goodman R, *et al* (2000) *The Mental Health of Children and Adolescents in Great Britain*. London: The Stationery Office.

58   Berelowitz M & Nelki J (1993) **Clinical syndromes in middle childhood**. In *Seminars in Child and Adolescent Psychiatry* (eds D Black & D Cottrell), pp. 124–153. London: Gaskell.

59   Costello E J (1998) cited in Wallace WA, Crown J M, Berger M, *et al* (1997) **Child and adolescent mental health: Health care needs assessment**. In *The Epidemiologically Based Needs Assessment Reviews* (eds A Stevens & J Raftery). 2nd series. Oxon: Radcliffe Medical Press Ltd.

60   Meltzer H, Gatward R, Goodman R, *et al* (2000) *The Mental Health of Children and Adolescents in Great Britain*. London: The Stationery Office.

61   World Health Organization (1992) *The ICD–10 Classification of Mental and Behavioural Disorders. Clinical Descriptions and Diagnostic Guidelines*. Geneva: WHO.

62   Klein R G (1994) **Anxiety disorders**. In *Child and Adolescent psychiatry: Modern Approaches* (eds M Rutter, E Taylor & L Hersov). 3rd edn. Oxford: Blackwell Scientific Publications.

63   American Psychiatric Association (2000) *Diagnostic and Statistical Manual of Mental Disorders*. 4th edn (DSM–IV–TR). Washington DC: APA.

The development of deliberate strategies to develop 'emotional literacy'[64] in children and adolescents should prevent some disorders and make others easier to treat. For a basic reference source, see Goleman (1995).[65] There is also a charity called 'Antidote', which promotes emotional literacy and produces an interesting newsletter with up-to-date news.[66]

What are the key messages from new research that are not being widely used?

Not enough use is made of existing psychoeducational materials about anxiety that can be given to parents and children.[67]

REFERENCES

● CLINICAL EVIDENCE ●

Panic disorder has been commissioned for future editions.

● SYSTEMATIC REVIEWS AND META-ANALYSES ●

Allen A J, Leonard H & Swedo S E (1995) **Current knowledge of medications for treatment of childhood anxiety disorders**. *Journal of the American Academy of Child and Adolescent Psychiatry*, **34**, 976–986.

Estrada A & Pinsof W (1995) **The effectiveness of family therapies for selected behavioural disorders of childhood**. *Journal of Marital and Family Therapy*, **21**, 403–440.

Fawcett J & Barkin R L (1998) **A meta-analysis of eight randomized, double-blind, controlled clinical trials of mirtazapine for the treatment of patients with major depression and symptoms of anxiety**. *Journal of Clinical Psychiatry*, **59**, 123–127.

Gammans R E, Stringfellow J C, Hvizdos A J, *et al* (1992) **Use of busprione in patients with generalized anxiety disorder and coexisting depressive symptoms: a meta-analysis of eight randomized, controlled studies**. *Neuropsychobiology*, **25**, 193–201.

Gerlsman C, Emmelkamp P M & Arrindell W A (1990) **Anxiety, depression, and perception of early parenting: a meta-analysis**. *Clinical Psychology Review*, **10**, 251–277. (Erratum: **11**, 667).

Kendall P & Treadwell K (1996) **Cognitive behavioural treatment for childhood anxiety disorders**. In *Psychosocial Treatments for Child and Adolescent Disorders: Empirically Based Strategies for Clinical Practice* (eds E Hibbs & P Jensen). Washington DC: APA.

---

64   See, for example, Whitfield R, *Life Foundations*. £95.00. Tel: 01279 442529.
65   Goleman D (1995) *Emotional Intelligence*. New York: Bantam Books.
66   Antidote, 5th Floor, 45 Beech Street, London EC2 8AD.
67   O'Neill C (1993) *Relax*. Child's Play (International) Ltd. ISBN 0-85953-79-7. A book for younger children that teaches how to recognise the symptoms of anxiety and ways to relax the mind and body.
       Lori Lite (1996) **A Boy and a Bear – The Children's Relaxation Book**. Speciality Press Inc. ISBN 1-886941-07-4. This book for 3–10-year-olds teaches young children how to relax to reduce anxiety and improve self-confidence.
       Young Minds (1996) *Mental Health in Your School*. London: Jessica Kingsley. £6.95.

Mendes H A, Lima M S & Hotopf M H (2000) **Serotonin reuptake inhibitors and new generation antidepressants for panic disorder**. Protocol for Cochrane Review. In *The Cochrane Library*, Issue 4. Oxford: Update Software.

Oosterlaan J, Logan G D & Sergeant J A (1998) **Response inhibition in AD/HD, CD, comorbid AD/HD + CD, anxious, and control children: a meta-analysis of studies with the stop task**. *Journal of Child Psychology and Psychiatry*, **39**, 411–425.

Petruzzello S J, Landers D M, Hatfield B D, *et al* (1991) **A meta-analysis on the anxiety-reducing effects of acute and chronic exercise. Outcomes and mechanisms**. *Sports Medicine*, **11**, 143–182.

Remschmidt H (1973) **Observations on the role of anxiety in neurotic and psychotic disorders at an early age**. *Journal of Autism and Childhood Schizophrenia*, **3**, 106–114.

Timberlake E M (1984) **Psychosocial functioning of school phobics at follow-up**. *Social Work Research and Abstracts*, **20**, 13–18.

● PRACTICE PARAMETERS ●

American Academy of Child and Adolescent Psychiatry (1997) **Practice parameters for the assessment and treatment of children with anxiety disorders**. *Journal of American Academy of Child and Adolescent Psychiatry*, **36** (suppl.), 69–84.

● REVIEWS ●

Bernstein G A, Borchardt C M & Perwien A R (1996) **Anxiety disorders in children and adolescents: a review of the past ten years**. *Journal of the American Academy of Child and Adolescent Psychiatry*, **35**, 110–119.

● CLASSIC PAPERS ●

Barlow D H, Cohen A S, Waddel M, *et al* (1984) **Panic and generalized anxiety disorders: nature and treatment**. *Behavior Therapy*, **15**, 431–449.

Dadds M, Heard P & Rapee R (1992) **The role of family intervention in the treatment of anxiety disorders: Some preliminary findings**. *Behaviour Change*, **9**, 171–177.

Graziano A M & Mooney K C (1982) **Behavioural treatment of 'nightfears' in children: Maintenance of improvement at 2½–3 year follow-up**. *Journal of Consulting Clinical Psychology*, **50**, 598–599.

● CUTTING EDGE PAPERS ●

Barrett P M, Dadds M R & Rapee R M (1996) **Family treatment of childhood anxiety: a controlled trial**. *Journal of Consulting and Clinical Psychology*, **64**, 333–342.

Kendall P C, Flannery-Schroeder E, Panichelli-Mindel S M, *et al* (1997) **Therapy for youths with anxiety disorders: a second randomized clinical trial**. *Journal of Consulting and Clinical Psychology*, **65**, 366–380.

King N J & Ollendick T H (1997) **Annotation: Treatment of childhood phobias**. *Journal of Child Psychology and Psychiatry*, **38**, 389–400.

● BOOKS ●

Blagg N (1987) *School Phobia and its Treatment*. London: Croom Helm.

—— (1999) **Fear and anxiety problems**. In *The Handbook of Child and Adolescent Clinical Psychology* (ed. A. Carr). London: Routledge.

Dwidevi K & Varma M (1997) *A Handbook of Childhood Anxiety Management*. Aldershot: Arena.

Husain S A & Kashani J H (1992) *Anxiety Disorders in Children and Adolescents*. Washington DC: American Psychiatric Press.

Kendall P C *et al* (1990) *Cognitive Behavioural Therapy for Anxious Children: A Treatment Manual*. Admore, PA: Workbook Publishing.

Ollendick T, King N & Yule W (1994) *International Handbook of Phobic and Anxiety Disorders in Children and Adolescents*. New York: Plenum.

Cochrane Controlled Trials Register
22 hits (keywords: phobia* AND child*)
180 hits (keywords: child* AND anxiety disorder*)

Cochrane Depression, Anxiety and Neurosis Group
Contact: Dr Natalie Khin, Review Group Coordinator, New Zealand.
n.khin@auckland.ac.nz

EMOTIONAL DISORDERS: depression

INTRODUCTION

Depression can be defined as depressed mood or loss of enjoyment plus three or four associated symptoms such as sleep disturbance, hopelessness and suicidality. The concept of depression in children has been controversial. It has only recently become more evident that children can exhibit depressive disorders similar to adults.

It has been argued that there are three main differences in depression in children compared with adults:

❍ There are developmental issues that relate to the age differences in the presence of affective symptoms.

❍ Children have different cognitive abilities and this will give rise to differences in their experience of the cognitive features that are associated with adult depression.

❍ To apply adult criteria to children assumes that they are able to accurately report their experience of depression.[68]

Depressive disorder is very uncommon in pre-pubertal children, but markedly increases in prevalence during early to mid-adolescence. The ONS survey estimates that depression occurs in 0.2% of boys and 0.3% of girls between the ages of 5 and 10 years and 1.7% of boys and 1.9% of girls between the ages of 11 and 15 years.[69]

DIAGNOSIS AND AETIOLOGY

The criteria for diagnosis of depression in children and adolescents is the same as the diagnosis for adults in both the ICD–10 and the DSM–IV–TR.

Depressive symptoms are very common in adolescents and depression should therefore only be diagnosed when the following are present:

❍ significantly impaired social functioning;

❍ psychopathological symptoms such as a suicide attempt; and

❍ significant suffering from the symptoms.

The aetiological factors of depressive disorder in young people appear to be related to early adverse experiences and certain temperamental features. These factors may predispose young people to develop depression, especially in those genetically at risk.

CRITICAL QUESTIONS

by Professor Richard Harrington and Dr Ann York

What developments have there been in the management of depression in the past 2–5 years?

Professor Richard Harrington   There is now good evidence for a modest genetic component for depressive symptoms in adolescence, although it is not yet clear

68   Harrington R (1994) **Affective disorders**. In *Child and Adolescent Psychiatry: Modern Approaches* (eds M Rutter, E Taylor & L Hersov). London: Blackwell Scientific Publications.
69   Meltzer H, Gatward R, Goodman R, *et al* (2000) *The Mental Health of Children and Adolescents in Great Britain*. London: The Stationery Office.

whether the results apply to depression as a disorder. Genetic effects appear to be indirect to the extent that they either increase the likelihood of experiencing adversity or alter the adolescent's reaction to adversity.

It has also become clear that tricyclic antidepressants are not an effective treatment for depression in either children or adolescents. There have been encouraging preliminary results with selective serotonin reuptake inhibitors (SSRIs), but the results of a large early trial require replication. There is now substantial evidence that cognitive–behavioural therapy (CBT) is an effective form of treatment for moderately severe depression in adolescents. However, it is still not clear how severe depression is best managed.

Dr Ann York   We are beginning to unravel more about what makes depression likely to persist. Family dysfunction, a poor relationship between mother and partner, severely disappointing events for the adolescents and poor friendships have been shown to predict persistence. Clinically, this points the way to further research into the impact of the treatment on these factors and how this influences the course and persistence of the depression. More research is needed into interpersonal psycho-therapy and family therapy as treatments for depression in children and adolescents. We also do not yet know how long to give treatment, whether combinations of treatment have additional, addictive effects, which components of CBT are responsible for the therapeutic effect and which treatments work for whom.

What are the key messages from new research that are not being widely used?

Dr Ann York   Major depressive disorder frequently goes undetected, especially in adolescents. Improvements are needed in the training of both multi-disciplinary child and adolescent services (CAMHS) professionals and Tier 1 workers, such as social workers, teachers and general practitioners.

Despite evidence from meta-analysis that CBT is a beneficial treatment for children and adolescents with depression (mainly those with mild to moderate depression), many young people are not able to receive this form of treatment owing to lack of trained staff in CAMHS. Randomised controlled trials have not yet demonstrated that family therapy is as effective as CBT for the treatment of depression in young people, yet clinically this may be the most frequently used treatment. It may, however, be helpful for comorbid conditions and in facilitating remission following CBT – more research is needed.

Depressive disorder is associated with suicidal ideation, suicide attempts and completed suicide and predicts subsequent ideation and attempts. Clinicians need to ensure that they enquire specifically about mood disorders in the assessment of deliberate self-harm in young people, although as yet it is not clear whether treatment of depression reduces suicide.

REFERENCES

● CLINICAL EVIDENCE ●

Hazell P (2000) **Depression in children and adolescents**. In *Clinical Evidence: A Compendium of the Best Available Evidence for Effective Health Care*, Issue 4, pp. 536–542. London: BMJ Publishing Group.

● SYSTEMATIC REVIEWS AND META-ANALYSES ●

Angold A, Costello E J & Erkanli A (1999) **Comorbidity**. *Journal of Child Psychology and Psychiatry*, **40**, 57–87.

Beasley C M (Jr), Dornseif B E, Bosomworth J C, *et al* (1991) **Fluoxetine and suicide: A meta-analysis of controlled trials for depression**. *British Medical Journal*, **303**, 685–692.

Beck C T (1998) **The effects of postpartum depression on child development: a meta-analysis**. *Archives of Psychiatric Nursing*, **12**, 12–20.

Bennett D S (1994) **Depression among children with chronic medical problems: a meta-analysis**. *Journal of Paediatric Psychology*, **19**, 149–169.

Berg A, Dencker K & Skarsatter I (1992) *Evidence-Based Nursing in the Treatment of People with Depression*. Swedish Council for Technology Assessment in Health Care (SBU), Swedish Nurses Association (SSF). Report No. 3, 9187890577. (Reviewed on Cochrane's Health Technology Assessment Database.)

Biederman J, Gonzalez E, Bronstein B, *et al* (1998) **Desipramine and cutaneous reactions in pediatric outpatients**. *Journal of Clinical Psychiatry*, **49**, 178–183.

Braun C M, Larocque C, Daigneault S, *et al* (1999) **Mania, pseudomania, depression, and pseudodepression resulting from focal unilateral cortical lesions**. *Neuropsychiatry, Neuropsychology and Behavior Neurology*, **12**, 35–51.

Churchill R, Wessely S & Lewis G (2000) **Pharmacotherapy and psychotherapy for depression**. Protocol for Cochrane Review. In *The Cochrane Library*, Issue 4. Oxford: Update Software.

Fawcett J & Barkin R L (1998) **A meta-analysis of eight randomized, double-blind, controlled clinical trials of mirtazapine for the treatment of patients with major depression and symptoms of anxiety**. *Journal of Clinical Psychiatry*, **59**, 123–127.

Gerlsma C, Emmelkamp P M & Arrindell W A (1990) **Anxiety, depression, and perception of early parenting: A meta-analysis**. *Clinical Psychology Review*, **10**, 251–277.

—, — & — (1991) **Anxiety, depression, and perception of early parenting: A meta-analysis: Erratum**. *Clinical Psychology Review*, **11**, 667.

Gladstone T R & Kaslow N J (1995) **Depression and attributions in children and adolescents: a meta-analysis**. *Journal of Abnormal Child Psychology*, **23**, 597–606.

Harrington R, Campbell F, Shoebridge P, *et al* (1998) **Meta-analysis of CBT for depression in adolescents**. *Journal of the American Academy of Child and Adolescent Psychiatry*, **37**, 1005–1006.

—, Whittaker J & Shoebridge P (1998) **Psychological treatment of depression in children and adolescents: A review of treatment research**. *British Journal of Psychiatry*, **173**, 291–298. (Review on DARE.)

—, —, —, *et al* (1998) **Systematic review of efficacy of cognitive behaviour therapies in child and adolescent depressive disorder**. *British Medical Journal*, **316**, 1559–1563. (Reviewed on DARE).

Hazell P, O'Connell D, Heathcote D, *et al* (1995) **Efficacy of tricyclic drugs in treating child and adolescent depression: a meta-analysis**. *British Medical Journal*, **310**, 897–901.

—, —, —, *et al* (2000) **Tricyclic drugs for depression in children and adolescents**. Cochrane Review. In *The Cochrane Library*, Issue 4. Oxford: Update Software.

Joiner T E & Wagner K D (1995) **Attribution style and depression in children and adolescents: A meta-analytic review**. *Clinical Psychology Review*, **15**, 777–798. (Reviewed on DARE.)

Lapalme M, Hodgins S & LaRoche C (1997) **Children of parents with bipolar disorder: a meta-analysis of risk for mental disorders**. *Canadian Journal of Psychiatry*, **42**, 623–631.

Marcotte D (1997) **Treating depression in adolescence: A review of the effectiveness of cognitive–behavioral treatments**. *Journal of Youth and Adolescence*, **26**, 273–283. (Reviewed on DARE.)

Patten S B (1991) **The loss of a parent during childhood as a risk factor for depression**. *Canadian Journal of Psychiatry*, **36**, 706–711.

Piccinin B & Ansseau M (1991) **Value of sleep and neuroendocrine tests as biological markers of depression in children and adolescents**. *Encephale*, **17**, 457–466.

Reinecke M A, Ryan N E & DuBois D L (1998) **Cognitive–behavioral therapy of depression and depressive symptoms during adolescence: A review and meta-analysis**. *Journal of the American Academy of Child and Adolescent Psychiatry*, **37**, 26–34. (Reviewed on DARE.)

—, — & — (1998) **Meta-analysis of CBT for depression in adolescents: Dr Reinecke *et al* reply**. *Journal of the American Academy of Child and Adolescent Psychiatry*, **37**, 1006–1007.

Thurber S, Ensign J, Punnett A F, *et al* (1995) **A meta-analysis of antidepressant outcome studies that involved children and adolescents**. *Journal of Clinical Psychology*, **51**, 340–345.

● PRACTICE PARAMETERS ●

American Academy of Child and Adolescent Psychiatry (1998) **Practice parameters for the assessment and treatment of children and adolescents with depressive disorders**. *Journal of the American Academy of Child and Adolescent Psychiatry*, **37** (suppl.), 63S–83S.

● CLINICAL GUIDELINES ●

Park R J & Goodyer I M (2000) **Clinical guidelines for depressive disorders in childhood and adolescence**. *European Journal of Child and Adolescent Psychiatry*, **9**, 147–161.

● REVIEWS ●

Devane C L & Sallee F R (1996) **Serotonin selective reuptake inhibitors in child and adolescent psychopharmacology: a review of published experience**. *Journal of Clinical Psychiatry*, **57**, 55–66.

Flemming J E & Offord D R (1990) **Epidemiology of childhood depressive disorders: A critical review**. *Journal of the American Academy of Child and Adolescent Psychiatry*, **29**, 571–580.

Flisher A J (1999) **Annotation: Mood disorder in suicidal children and adolescents: Recent development**. *Journal of Psychology and Psychiatry*, **40**, 315–324.

Walter G, Rey J M & Mitchell P B (1999) **Electroconvulsive therapy in adolescents**. *Journal of Child Psychology and Psychiatry*, **40**, 325–334.

● CLASSIC PAPERS ●

Harrington R, Fudge H, Rutter M, *et al* (1990) **Adult outcomes of childhood and adolescent depression: psychiatric status**. *Archives of General Psychiatry*, **47**, 465–473.

Kovacs M (1996) **Presentation and course of major depressive disorder during childhood and later years of the lifespan**. *Journal of the American Academy of Child and Adolescent Psychiatry*, **35**, 705–715.

Puig-Antich J, Lukens E, Davies M, *et al* (1985) **Psychosocial functioning in prepubertal major depressive disorders. Interpersonal relationships during the depressive episode**. *Archives of General Psychiatry*, **42**, 500–507.

——, Perel J M, Lupatkin W, *et al* (1987) **Imipramine in prepubertal major depressive disorders**. *Archives of General Psychiatry*, **44**, 81–89.

Rutter M (1986) **The developmental psychopathology of depression: issues and perspectives**. In *Depression in Young People: Developmental and Clinical Perspectives* (eds M Rutter, C Izard & P Read), pp. 3–30. New York: Guilford Press.

Ryan N D, Puig-Antich J, Ambrosini P, *et al* (1987) **The clinical picture of major depression in children and adolescents**. *Archives of General Psychiatry*, **44**, 854–861.

● CUTTING EDGE PAPERS ●

Angold A, Costello E, Erkanli A, *et al* (1999) **Pubertal changes in hormone levels and depression in girls**. *Psychological Medicine*, **29**, 1043–1053.

Brent D, Holder D, Kolko D, *et al* (1997) **A clinical psychotherapy trial for adolescent depression comparing cognitive, family and supportive treatments**. *Archives of General Psychiatry*, **54**, 877–885.

——, Kolko D J, Birmaher B, *et al* (1998) **Predictors of treatment efficacy in a clinical trial of three psychosocial treatments for adolescent depression**. *Journal of the American Academy of Child and Adolescent Psychiatry*, **37**, 906–914.

Eley T C, Deater-Deckard K & Fombonne E (1999) **An adoption study of depressive symptoms in middle childhood**. *Journal of Child Psychology and Psychiatry*, **39**, 337–345.

Emslie G, Rush A, Weinberg W, *et al* (1997) **A double-blind, randomized placebo-controlled trial of fluoxetine in depressed children and adolescents**. *Archives of General Psychiatry*, **54**, 1031–1037.

Goodyer I M, Herbert J, Secher S M, *et al* (1997) **Short-term outcome of major depression: comorbidity and severity at presentation as predictors of persistent disorder I**. *Journal of the American Academy of Child and Adolescent Psychiatry*, **36**, 179–187.

——, ——, Tamplin A, *et al* (1997) **Short-term outcome of major depression: life events, family dysfunction, and friendship difficulties as predictors of persistent disorder II**. *Journal of the American Academy of Child and Adolescent Psychiatry*, **36**, 474–480.

Hankin B L, Abramson L Y, Moffitt T E, *et al* (1998) **Development of depression from preadolescence to young adulthood: emerging gender differences in a 10-year longitudinal study**. *Journal of Abnormal Psychology*, **107**, 128–140.

Sapolsky R M (2000) **Gluco corticoids and hippocampal atrophy in neuro-psychiatric disorders**. *Archives of General Psychiatry*, **57**, 925–935.

Strober M, Rao U, De Antonio M, *et al* (1998) **Effects of electroconvulsive therapy in adolescents with severe endogenous depression resistant to pharmacotherapy**. *Biological Psychiatry*, **43**, 335–338.

● BOOKS ●

Goodyer I (ed.) (1995) *The Depressed Child and Adolescent. Developmental and Clinical Perspectives*. Cambridge: Cambridge University Press.

Harrington R C (1993) *Depressive Disorder in Childhood and Adolescence*. Chichester: Wiley.

● OTHER SOURCES ●

Aisher A J (1999) **Mood disorder in suicidal children and adolescents: recent developments**. *Journal of Child Psychology and Psychiatry*, **40**, 315–324.

Churchill R & Gill D (1996) **Drug treatment of childhood depression**. *Bandolier*, **3**, 29–37.

Weismann M M, Wolk S, Goldstein R B, *et al* (1999) **Depressed adolescents grown up**. *Journal of the American Academy of Child and Adolescent Psychiatry*, **281**, 1707–1713.

Cochrane Controlled Trials Register
50 hits (keywords: "childhood depression")
139 hits (keywords: "depressive disorder*" AND child*)
677 hits (keywords: "depressive disorder*" AND adolescen*)

Cochrane Depression, Anxiety and Neurosis Group
Contact: Dr Natalie Khin, Review Group Coordinator, New Zealand.
n.khin@auckland.ac.nz

INTRODUCTION

Obsessive–compulsive disorder (OCD) is characterised by repetitive and intrusive thoughts (obsessions) and/or rituals (compulsions) that cause distress and interfere with daily functioning. Usually, the person recognises that the obsessions/compulsions are irrational. However, this may not apply to children as they may not have the cognitive ability to reach this judgement.

OCD has been reported to occur in 1.9% of adolescents.[70] Boys tend to have an earlier onset of symptoms than girls, particularly before the age of seven years.[71]

DIAGNOSIS AND AETIOLOGY

The DSM–IV–TR and the ICD–10 diagnoses of OCD differ only slightly in their classification of the disorder.

The ICD–10 diagnosis focuses on the balance of obsessions or compulsions. There are four categories: predominantly obsessional thoughts or ruminations; predominantly compulsive acts; mixed obsessional thoughts/acts; obsessive–compulsive disorder unspecified/other obsessive–compulsive disorders. The DSM–IV–TR does not make this distinction and only distinguishes between obsessive–compulsive disorder of the normal type and obsessive–compulsive disorder with poor insight (inability to recognise that the obsessions or compulsions are excessive or unreasonable).

OCD appears to have some genetic basis, with 5% of parents having the disorder themselves and approximately two-thirds of parents having obsessional traits.[72]

OCD is estimated to occur in 0.1% of children between the ages of 5 and 10 years and in 0.5% of children between the ages of 11 and 15 years.[73]

CRITICAL QUESTIONS

by Dr Derek Bolton

What new developments have there been in the management of obsessive–compulsive disorder in the past 2–5 years?

While there is accumulating evidence of a genetic contribution to OCD, there has been relatively less attention paid to environmental and psychosocial factors involved in the genesis of the disorder. In the past two years, however, several studies and models have been published on this issue from a developmental perspective and involving integration of psychosocial and neurobiological processes.[74]

70 Wallace W A, Crown J M, Berger M, *et al* (1997) **Child and adolescent mental health: Health care needs assessment**. In *The Epidemiologically Based Needs Assessment Reviews* (eds A Stevens & J Raftery). 2nd series. Oxon: Radcliffe Medical Press.

71 Rapoport J L, Swedo S & Leonard H (1994) **Obsessiv–compulsive disorder**. In *Child and Adolescent Psychiatry: Modern Approaches* (eds M Rutter, E Taylor & L Hersov). 3rd edn. Oxford: Blackwell Scientific Publications.

72 Berelowitz M & Nelki J (1993) **Clinical syndrome in middle childhood**. In *Seminars in child and Adolescent Psychiatry* (eds D Black & D Cottrell), pp. 124–153. London: Gaskell.

73 Meltzer H, Gatward R, Goodman R, *et al* (2000) *The Mental Health of Children and Adolescents in Great Britain*. London: The Stationery Office.

74 e.g. Dinn W M, Harris C L & Raynard RC (1999) **Posttraumatic obsessive–compulsive disorder: a three-factor model**. *Psychiatry*, **63**, 313–324; Pollock R A & Carter A S (1999) **The familial and developmental context of obsessive–compulsive disorder**. *Child and Adolescent Psychiatric*

Treatment resistance and relapse following good treatment outcome remain outstanding issues. Most work on these problems has been done with adults, on two fronts: first, augmentation of SSRIs with other agents,[75] and second, in new cognitive models of the disorder.[76]

What are the key messages from new research that are not being widely used?

Evidence for the effectiveness of CBT, specifically including exposure with response-prevention, for OCD in adults has long been available, although so far there has been only one published randomised controlled evaluation of this treatment with children and adolescents, comparing with clomipramine.[77] These findings together with several recent published uncontrolled trials for the younger age groups strongly suggest that CBT including exposure with response-prevention is a clear treatment of choice for OCD in children and adolescents, as proposed in current practice parameters of the American Academy of Child and Adolescent Psychiatry (1998). However, these guidelines go on to remark: "One of the greatest barriers to successful CBT is the relative lack of psychotherapists trained in the method."[78] This point may apply less in the UK than the USA.

REFERENCES

● SYSTEMATIC REVIEWS AND META-ANALYSES ●

Brynska A & Wolanczyk T (1998) **Psychotherapeutic methods in the treatment of obsessive–compulsive disorder (OCD) in children and adolescents (in Polish)**. *Psychiatr. Pol.*, **32**, 723–738.

Geller D, Biederman J, Jones J, *et al* (1998) **Is juvenile obsessive–compulsive disorder a developmental subtype of the disorder? A review of the pediatric literature**. *Journal of the American Academy of Child and Adolescent Psychiatry*, **37**, 420–427.

Greist J H (1995) **Efficacy and tolerability of serotonin transport inhibitors in obsessive–compulsive disorder. A meta-analysis**. *Archives of General Psychiatry*, **52**, 53–60.

Neudorfl A & Herpertz-Dahlmann B (1996) **Follow-up of obsessive–compulsive disorders in childhood and adolescence: A review of the literature**. *Zeitschrift für Kinder- und Jugendpsychiatrie*, **24**, 105–116.

Clinics of North America, **8**, 461–479; Leckman J F, Mayes L C, Feldman R, *et al* (1999) Early parental preoccupations and behaviors and their possible relationship to the symptoms of obsessive–compulsive disorder. *Acta Psychiatrica Scandinavica*, **100** (suppl. 396), 1–26.

75 McDougle C J (1997) Update on pharmacologic management of OCD: agents and augmentation. *Journal of Clinical Psychiatry*, **58** (suppl. 12), 11–17; see also Rapoport J L & Inoff-Germain G (2000) Practitioner review: treatment of obsessive compulsive disorder in children and adolescents. *Journal of Child Psychology and Psychiatry*, **41**, 419–431.

76 Salkovskis P M (1999) Understanding and treating obsessive compulsive disorder. *Behaviour Research and Therapy*, **37**, S29–S52.

77 de Haan E, Hoogduin K, Buitelaar J, *et al* (1998) Behavior therapy versus clomipramine in obsessive compulsive disorder in children and adolescence. *Journal of the American Academy of Child and Adolescent Psychiatry*, **37**, 1022–1029.

78 American Academy of Child and Adolescent Psychiatry (1998) Practice parameters for the assessment and treatment of children and adolescents with obsessive–compulsive disorder. *Journal of the American Academy of Child and Adolescent Psychiatry*, **37** (suppl.), S35.

Piccinelli M, Pini S, Bellantuono C, *et al* (1995) **Efficacy of drug treatment in obsessive–compulsive disorder. A meta-analytic review**. *British Journal of Psychiatry*, **166**, 424–443. (Reviewed on DARE.)

Soomro G M, Oakley-Browne M & Doughty C (2000) **Serotonin re-uptake inhibitors (SSRIs) versus placebo for obsessive compulsive disorders**. Protocol for Cochrane Review. In *The Cochrane Library*, Issue 4. Oxford: Update Software.

● PRACTICE PARAMETERS ●

American Academy of Child and Adolescent Psychiatry (1998) **Practice parameters for the assessment and treatment of children and adolescents with obsessive–compulsive disorder**. *Journal of the American Academy of Child and Adolescent Psychiatry*, **37** (suppl. 10), 27S–45S.

● CLINICAL GUIDELINES ●

March J, Frances A, Carpenter D, *et al* (1997) **The expert consensus guideline series: treatment of obsessive–compulsive disorder**. *Journal of Clinical Psychiatry*, **4** (suppl.), 2–72.

Thomsen P H (1998) **Obsessive–compulsive disorder in children and adolescents. Clinical guidelines**. *European Child and Adolescent Psychiatry*, **7**, 1–11.

● REVIEWS ●

Bolton D (1998) **Obsessive compulsive disorder**. In *Comprehensive Clinical Psychology*, Vol. 5 (eds M Hersen & A Bellack), pp. 367–391. San Francisco, CA: Pergamon.

Goodman W (1999) **Obsessive compulsive disorder: diagnosis and treatment**. *Journal of Clinical Psychiatry*, **60** (suppl. 18), 27–32.

Rapoport J L & Inoff-Germain G (2000) **Practitioner review: treatment of obsessive compulsive disorder in children and adolescents**. *Journal of Child Psychology and Psychiatry*, **41**, 419–431.

Salkovskis P M (1999) **Understanding and treating obsessive compulsive disorder**. *Behaviour Research and Therapy*, **37**, S29–S52.

● CLASSIC PAPERS ●

Bolton D, Collins S & Steinberg D (1983) **The treatment of obsessive-compulsive disorder in adolescence: a report of fifteen cases**. *British Journal of Psychiatry*, **142**, 456–464.

Leonard H L, Swedo S E, Rapoport J L, *et al* (1989) **Treatment of obsessive-compulsive disorder with clomipramine and desipramine in children and adolescents**. *Archives of General Psychiatry*, **46**, 1088–1092.

Valleni-Basile L A, Garrison C Z, Jackson K L, *et al* (1994) **Frequency of obsessive-compulsive disorder in a community sample of young adolescents**. *Journal of the American Academy of Child and Adolescent Psychiatry*, **33**, 782–791.

● CUTTING EDGE PAPERS ●

De Haan E, Hoogduin K, Buitelaar J, *et al* (1998) **Behavior therapy versus clomipramine in obsessive compulsive disorder in children and adolescence**. *Journal of the American Academy of Child and Adolescent Psychiatry*, **37**, 1022–1029.

Swedo S E, Leonard H L, Garvey M, *et al* (1998) **Pediatric autoimmune neuropsychiatric disorders associated with streptococcal infections: Clinical description of the first 50 cases**. *American Journal of Psychiatry*, **155**, 264–271.

● BOOKS ●

March J & Mulle K (1998) *OCD in Children and Adolescents: A Cognitive Behavioural Treatment Manual*. New York: Guilford Press.

● USEFUL WEBSITES ●

Obsessive Compulsive Disorder (OCD) Resources Centre http://ocd resource.com

---

Cochrane Controlled Trials Register
63 hits (keywords: "obsessive compulsive disorder" AND child*)
105 hits (keywords: "obsessive compulsive disorder" AND adolescence)
42 hits (keywords: "obsessive compulsive disorder" AND adolescent*)

Cochrane Depression, Anxiety and Neurosis Group
Contact: Dr Natalie Khin, Review Group Coordinator, New Zealand.
n.khin@auckland.ac.nz

GENDER IDENTITY DISORDERS

INTRODUCTION

Gender identity disorders are characterised by a strong and persistent cross-gender identification where the child has a persistent desire to be of the other sex.[79] Some children may refuse to attend school because of teasing or may feel isolated because of the failure to develop age-appropriate, same-sex peer relationships.

Gender identity disorders manifest differently across the lifecycle. These disorders tend to be more common in males than females. It is estimated that the prevalence of gender identity disorders is 3–4%,[80] and that one- to two-thirds of boys with gender identity disorder of childhood will show homosexual orientation during and after adolescence.[81]

DIAGNOSIS AND AETIOLOGY

The ICD–10 category of adult personality and behaviour has a broad category of gender identity disorders in which there is a category for gender identity disorder of childhood. This diagnosis can only be made before the onset of puberty.

Under the category sexual and gender identity disorders, the DSM–IV–TR has two categories of gender identity disorder based on the current age of the person. These two categories are gender identity disorder in children and gender identity disorder in adolescence or adults.

CRITICAL QUESTIONS

by Dr Domenico Di Ceglie

What new developments have there been in the management of gender identity disorders in the past 2–5 years?

In the past few years, more integrated and comprehensive management plans have been developed for children, and particularly adolescents, with gender identity disorders. This model, which includes a combination of psychological, social and physical intervention, could be defined as the 'staged approach'.

- ❍ Stage 1: this involves psychological exploration with the child/adolescent and the family as well as psychosocial interventions.

- ❍ Stage 2: for adolescents who are evolving towards transsexualism, reversible physical interventions such as the use of hypothalamic blockers may be considered.

- ❍ Stage 3: during late adolescence, partially reversible interventions, such as the use of hormone treatment, can be considered.

---

79 Le Couteur A (1993) **Clinical syndromes in early childhood**. In *Seminars in Child and Adolescent Psychiatry* (eds D Black & D Cottrell), pp. 95–123. London: Gaskell.
American Psychiatric Association (2000) *Diagnostic and Statistical Manual of Mental Disorders*. 4th edn (DSM–IV–TR). Washington DC: APA.

80 Le Couteur A (1993) **Clinical syndromes in early childhood**. In *Seminars in Child and Adolescent Psychiatry* (eds D Black & D Cottrell), pp. 95–123. London: Gaskell.

81 World Health Organization (1992) *The ICD–10 Classification of Mental and Behavioural Disorders: Clinical Descriptions and Diagnostic Guidelines*. Geneva: WHO.

○ Stage 4: irreversible interventions are considered only in adulthood after the age of 18 years.

Within this framework, some children and adolescents may progress from one stage to the next with some interventions from the previous stage continuing, while others may wish to stop at a particular stage of the process.

This framework also provides a containing function for intense feelings of anxiety and despair that teenagers in particular may present.[82]

What are the key messages from new research that are not being widely used?

A follow-up study of transsexual adolescents who, after careful assessment, started the process of sex reassignment during adolescence (after the age of 16 years) shows that they had achieved a good level of psychological and social adjustment at least one year after surgical intervention.[83] However, further outcome research is needed.

REFERENCES

● SYSTEMATIC REVIEWS AND META-ANALYSES ●

Di Ceglie D (2000) **Gender identity disorder in young people**. *Advances in Psychiatric Treatment*, **6**, 458–466.

Murnen S K & Smolak L (1997) **Femininity, masculinity, and disordered eating: a meta-analytic review**. *International Journal of Eating Disorders*, **22**, 231–242.

Scott Heller S (1997) **Gender identity disorder**. *The Signal – Newsletter of the World Association for Infant Mental Health*, **5**, 1–8.

Stevenson M R & Black K N (1988) *Paternal absence and sex-role development: a meta-analysis*. **Child Development**, **59**, 793–814.

● CLASSIC PAPERS ●

Coates S, Friedman R C & Wolfe S (1991) **The aetiology of boyhood gender identity disorder: a model for integrating temperament development and psychodynamics**. *Psychoanalytic Dialogues*, **1**, 481–523.

Money J (1994) **The concept of gender identity in childhood and adolescence after 39 years**. *Journal of Sex and Marital Therapy*, **20**, 163–177.

Stoller R J (1992) **Gender identity development and prognosis: a summary**. In ***New Approaches to Mental Health from Birth to Adolescence*** (eds C Chiland & J G Young), pp. 185–197. New Haven and London: Yale University Press.

● CUTTING EDGE PAPERS ●

Di Ceglie D (1998) **Management and therapeutic aims in working with children and adolescents with gender identity disorders, and their families**.

---

82 Di Ceglie D (2000) Gender identity disorder in young people. *Advances in Psychiatric Treatment*, 6, 458–466.
83 Cohen-Kettenis P T & van Goozen S M M (1997) **Sex ressaignment of adolescent transsexuals: a follow-up study**. *Journal of the American Academy of Child and Adolescent Psychiatry*, 36, 263–271.

In *A Stranger in My Own Body – Atypical Gender Identity Development and Mental Health* (eds D De Ceglie with D Freedman), pp. 185–197. London: Karnac Books.

Cohen-Kettenis P T & van Goozen S M M (1997) **Sex reassignment of adolescent transsexuals: a follow-up study**. *Journal of the American Academy of Child and Adolescent Psychiatry*, **36**, 263–271.

● REPORTS ●

Royal College of Psychiatrists (1998) *Gender Identity Disorders in Children and Adolescents: Guidance for Management*. Council Report CR63. London: Royal College of Psychiatrists.

● BOOKS ●

Di Ceglie D with Freedman D (eds) (1998) *A Stranger in My Own Body – Atypical Gender Identity Development and Mental Health*. London: Karnac Books.

Green R (1994) *Sexual Identity Conflicts in Children and Adolescents*. New York: Basic Books.

Zucker K J & Bradley S J (1995) *Gender Identity Disorders and Psychosexual Problems in Children and Adolescents*. New York: Guilford Press.

INTRODUCTION

Chronic fatigue syndrome is characterised by persistent and recurrent fatigue that is severe and disabling. Other symptoms include headaches, difficulty concentrating, sleep difficulties and musculoskeletal pain. The symptoms of chronic fatigue are not relieved by rest, and a noticeable reduction in previous levels of activity is evident.[84]

There do not seem to be any prevalence figures of chronic fatigue syndrome in children, however the presence of the disorder in the general population is estimated to be between 0.2% and 2.6%.[85]

DIAGNOSIS AND AETIOLOGY

For a diagnosis of chronic fatigue syndrome to be made, the ICD–10 requires the presence of mental fatigue, whereas the DSM–IV–TR requires the presence of severe physical symptoms. Aside from this difference, the two sets of criteria are comparable.

Children with chronic fatigue syndrome appear to have a fairly good prognosis. In a six-year follow-up study, 54–94% of children showed noticeable improvement.[86]

CRITICAL QUESTIONS

by Professor Simon Wessely and Professor Elena Garralda

What developments have there been in the management of chronic fatigue syndrome in the past 2–5 years?

Professor Simon Wessely   There are rarely great 'breakthroughs' in the field of chronic fatigue syndrome, rather a gradual re-emergence of clinical common sense. We still lack sufficient research on management and outcomes in children.

Professor Elena Garralda   There is a better understanding of the outcome of chronic fatigue syndrome with severe cases; for example, an illness duration of about three years, leading to recovery in two out of three cases, but a tendency to experience symptoms of fatigue of less intensity in half the recovered group. There also seem to be associated psychiatric disorders in at least half the affected subjects.

Audits of clinical practice and good recommendations for treatment have been published.[87]

What are the key messages from new research that are not being widely used?

Professor Simon Wessely   In general, there are still occasions on which clinicians continue to manage children without the support of a multi-disciplinary team or without knowledge of a bio-psychosocial approach, however, such instances are increasingly uncommon.

---

84   Reid S, Chalder T, Cleare A, *et al* (2000) Chronic fatigue syndrome. In *Clinical Evidence*, Issue 3, pp. 486–495. London: BMJ Publishing Group.

85   As above.

86   As above.

87   Garralda M E (ed.) (1999) *Chronic Fatigue Syndrome: Helping Children and Adolescents*. Occasional Paper 16. London: ACPP; Rangel L, Rapp S, Levin M, *et al* (1999) Chronic fatigue syndrome: updates on paediatric and psychological management. *Current Paediatrics*, **9**, 188–193.

Professor Elena Garralda   It is evident that it is essential to assess the full psychiatric state of affected subjects.

The development of specialist child and adolescent psychiatric units does not stem from research in the area, but from clinical practice.

REFERENCES

● CLINICAL EVIDENCE ●

Reid S, Chalder T, Cleare A, *et al* (2000) **Chronic fatigue syndrome**. In *Clinical Evidence: A Compendium of the Best Available Evidence for Effective Health Care*, Issue 4, pp. 578–586. London: BMJ Publishing Group.

● SYSTEMATIC REVIEWS AND META-ANALYSES ●

None identified.

● CLINICAL GUIDELINES ●

None identified.

● REVIEWS ●

Richards J (2000) **Chronic fatigue syndrome in children and adolescents: a review article**. *Clinical Child Psychology and Psychiatry*, **5**, 31–51.

Wright J B & Beverly D W (1998) **Chronic fatigue syndrome**. *Archives of Disease in Childhood*, **79**, 368–374.

● CLASSIC PAPERS ●

Bell K M, Cookfair D, Bell D S, *et al* (1991) **Risk factors associated with chronic fatigue syndrome in cluster of paediatric cases**. *Review of Infectious Disease*, **13** (suppl.), 32S–38S.

Vereker M (1992) **Chronic fatigue syndrome: a joint paediatric–psychiatric approach**. *Archives of Disease in Childhood*, **67**, 550–555.

Walford G A, Nelson W M & McCluskey D R (1993) **Fatigue, depression and social adjustment in chronic fatigue syndrome**. *Archives of Disease in Childhood*, **68**, 348–388.

Wessely S (1990) **Old wine in new bottles: neurasthenia and 'ME'**. *Psychological Medicine*, **20**, 35–53.

● CUTTING EDGE PAPERS ●

Carter B, Edwards J, Kronenberger W, *et al* (1995) **Case control study of chronic fatigue in paediatric patients**. *Pediatrics*, **95**, 179–186.

Fox R (1998) ***A Research Portfolio on Chronic Fatigue***. London: The Royal Society of Medicine Press.

Fry A & Martin M (1996) **Cognitive idiosyncrasies among children with the chronic fatigue syndrome: anomalies in self-reported activity levels**. *Journal of Psychosomatic Research*, **41**, 213–223.

Garralda M E, Rangel L A, Levin M, *et al* (1999) **Psychiatric adjustment in adolescents with a history of childhood chronic fatigue syndrome**. *Journal of the American Academy of Child and Adolescent Psychiatry*, **38**, 1515–1521.

Plioplys A (1997) **Chronic fatigue syndrome should not be diagnosed in children**. *Pediatrics*, **100**, 270–271.

Rangel L A, Garralda M E, Levin M, *et al* (2000) **The course of chronic fatigue syndrome**. *Journal of the Royal Society of Medicine*, **38**, 129–134.

——, ——, ——, *et al* (2000) **Personality in adolescents with chronic fatigue syndrome**. *European Child and Adolescent Psychiatry*, **9**, 39–45.

● REPORTS ●

Anon (1997 amended) *Chronic Fatigue Syndrome: Report of the Committee of the Royal Colleges of Physicians, Psychiatrists and General Practioners*. London: Royal College of Physicians.

Best L & Stevens A (1996) *Cognitive Behavioural Therapy in the Treatment of Chronic Fatigue Syndrome*. Development and Evaluation Committee (Report 50). Southampton: Wessex Institute for Health Research and Development. (Refers to all ages.)

Garralda M E (ed.) (1999) *Chronic Fatigue Syndrome: Helping Children and Adolescents*. Occasional Paper 16. London: ACPP.

● BOOKS ●

Marcovitch H (1991) *Chronic Fatigue States in Children*. In *Post Viral Fatigue Syndrome* (eds R Jenkins & J Mowbray), pp. 335–433. Chichester: John Wiley and Sons.

Taylor D (1992) *Outlandish Factitious Illness*. In *Recent Advances in Paediatrics* (ed. T David), pp. 63–76. Edinburgh: Churchill Livingstone.

Wessely S, Hotopf M & Sharpe M (1998) *Chronic Fatigue and its Syndromes*. Oxford: Oxford University Press.

Cochrane Controlled Trials Register
3 hits (keywords: chronic fatigue syndrome* AND child*)

Cochrane Depression, Anxiety and Neurosis Group
Contact: Dr Natalie Khin, Review Group Coordinator, New Zealand.
n.khin@auckland.ac.nz

INTRODUCTION

Dementia results from a disease of the brain in which many of the higher coritical functions such as memory, thinking, language, processing of information, reasoning and comprehension are affected. There is usually a decline in intellectual functioning that impacts on daily functioning.[88]

DIAGNOSIS AND AETIOLOGY

There is no category for dementia in children or adolescents in the ICD–10 or DSM–IV–TR.

REFERENCES

● REVIEWS ●

Goodman R (1994) *Brain Disorders*. In *Child and Adolescent Psychiatry: Modern Approaches* (eds M Rutter, E Taylor & L Hersov), pp. 172–190 (especially pp. 179–182). Oxford: Blackwell Scientific Publications.

88   World Health Organization (1992) *The ICD–10 Classification of Mental and Behavioural Disorders: Clinical Descriptions and Diagnostic Guidelines*. Geneva: WHO.

INTRODUCTION

Disintegrative disorder (or Heller's disease) refers to a condition with onset after the age of two years, where following a normal period of development, a child experiences massive skill loss or marked developmental regression. The resulting pattern of symptoms is similar to that of autism,[89] although it differs in that motor and self-help skills can be lost as well as some complex stereotyped behavioural patterns.[90]

The aetiology of the disorder is uncertain. Disintegrative disorder has been linked with measles encephalitis, cerebral lipoidoses, leukodystrophies and other neurological conditions, but usually it is difficult to find a direct cause of the disorder.[91]

The prognosis of the disorder appears to be worse than autism or other pervasive developmental disorders that have a late onset. There is some debate as to whether disintegrative disorder can be meaningfully distinguished from autism.[92]

REFERENCES

● REVIEWS ●

Harris J C (1996) **Childhood disintegrative disorder**. *Developmental Neuropsychiatry*, **2**, 239–243.

● CUTTING EDGE PAPERS ●

Russo M, Perry R, Kolodny E, *et al* (1996) **Heller syndrome in a pre-school boy. Proposed medical evaluation and hypothesized pathogenesis**. *European Child and Adolescent Psychiatry*, **5**, 172–177.

89   Evan-Jones L G & Rosenbloom L (1978) cited in Graham P (1991) **Development and its disorders**. In *Child Psychiatry: A Developmental Approach*, pp. 161–162. Oxford: Oxford University Press.
90   Lord C & Rutter M (1994) **Autism and pervasive developmental disorders**. In *Child and Adolescent Psychiatry: Modern Approaches* (eds M Rutter, Taylor E & L Hersov), pp. 569–593. London: Blackwell Scientific Publications.
91   As above.
92   Volkmar F R & Cohen D J (1989) cited in Graham P (1991) **Development and its disorders**. In *Child Psychiatry: A Developmental Approach*, pp. 161–162. Oxford: Oxford University Press.

INTRODUCTION

Down's syndrome is the most common genetic form of mental retardation. It is associated with impaired intellectual development as well as some degree of mental handicap.

Children with Down's syndrome have a characteristic facial appearance, with a smaller fronto-occipital diameter of the skull. They are also more at risk of developing congenital cardiac abnormalities, sensory impairments, respiratory disorders and leukaemia.[93]

Down's syndrome usually results from the inheritance of an extra chromosome (trisomy 21). Occasionally, Down's syndrome can also result from an unbalanced chromosomal translocation that can be inherited – this has a different recurrence risk than that of trisomy 21.[94]

Down's syndrome is estimated to occur in 1 in 600 births.[95]

REFERENCES

● REVIEWS ●

Johannsen P, Christensen J E & Mai J (1996) **The prevalence of dementia in Down syndrome**. *Dementia*, **7**, 221–225.

Zigman W B, Schupf N, Sersen E, *et al* (1996) **Prevalence of dementia in adults with and without Down syndrome**. *American Journal of Mental Retardation*, **100**, 403–412.

● USEFUL WEBSITES ●

Downs Syndrome Association http://dsa-uk.com

93   Bolton P & Holland A (1994) **Chromosomal abnormalities**. In *Child and Adolescent Psychiatry: Modern Approaches* (eds M Rutter, E Taylor & L Hersov). London: Blackwell Scientific Publications.
94   As above.
95   As above.

PAEDIATRIC LIAISON: Rett's syndrome

INTRODUCTION

Rett's syndrome is a progressive neurological disorder that only occurs in girls.

Typically, a girl will develop normally for the first 7–18 months, which is then followed by a period of developmental stagnation. Following this stage is a stage of rapid skill loss such that the child is left with a mental age of 6–9 months. A child with Rett's syndrome could remain at this mental age for years.[96]

Rett's syndrome results in limited use of the hands, impaired mobility, episodic hyperventilation, episodic laughter and a typically small head circumference.[97]

The aetiology of Rett's syndrome is unknown.

REFERENCES

● REVIEWS ●

Amir R E, Van den Veyver I B, Wan M, *et al* (1999) **Rett Syndrome is caused by mutations in X-linked MECP2, encoding methyl-CpG-binding protein 2**. *Nature Genetics*, **23**, 185–188.

Harris J C (1996) **Rett's disorder**. *Developmental Neuropsychiatry*, **2**, 228–238.

● CUTTING EDGE PAPERS ●

Leonard H & Bower C (1998) **Is the girl with Rett syndrome normal at birth?** *Developmental Medicine and Child Neurology*, **40**, 115–121.

---

96   Goodman R (1994) **Brain disorders**. In *Child and Adolescent Psychiatry: Modern Approaches* (eds M Rutter, E Taylor & L Hersov). London: Blackwell Scientific Publications.
97   As above.

INTRODUCTION

Subacute sclerosing panencephalitis is a gradual virus infection caused by the measles virus. The onset is between 5 and 15 years of age and often begins with intellectual deterioration and personality change. As the disorder progresses, a child will experience myoclonic jerks. Initially, these jerks are infrequent and could lead to falling, but as the jerks become more frequent (every 10–15 seconds) they can affect the whole body. The jerks seem to be aggravated by loud noises or excitement and are absent during sleep.[98]

Subacute sclerosing panencephalitis is five times more likely to occur in boys than in girls.[99]

REFERENCES

● REVIEWS ●

Gascon C G (1996) **Subacute sclerosing panencephalitis**. *Seminars in Pediatric Neurology*, **3**, 260–269.

● CUTTING EDGE PAPERS ●

Forrest G & Stores G (1996) **Subacute sclerosing panencephalitis presenting with psychosis and possible sexual abuse**. *European Child and Adolescent Psychiatry*, **5**, 110–113.

Papazian O, Canizales E, Alfonson I, *et al* (1995) **Reversible dementia and apparent brain atrophy during valporate therapy**. *Annals of Neurology*, **38**, 687–691.

Cochrane Controlled Trials Register
11 hits (keywords: "Rett syndrome")
1 hit (keywords: autism AND dementia)
6 hits (keywords: "down syndrome" AND dementia)
2 hits (keywords: "subacute sclerosing panencephalitis" AND child)

Cochrane Movement Disorders Group
Contact: Dr Joaquim Ferreire, Review Group Coordinator, Lisbon, Portugal.
Tel: +351 1797 3453. Movementdisord@mail.telepac.pt

---

98   Goodman R (1994) **Brain disorders**. In *Child and Adolescent Psychiatry: Modern Approaches* (eds M Rutter, E Taylor & L Hersov). London: Blackwell Scientific Publications.
99   As above.

INTRODUCTION

Somatoform disorders can be described as the presence of physical symptoms that cannot be linked to a physical illness. The types of symptoms that can occur are complete or partial paralyses, convulsions of the limbs, anaesthetic areas of the skin, visual difficulties, pains and fatigue.[100]

DIAGNOSIS AND AETIOLOGY

There is no specific category for the diagnosis of somatoform disorders for children and adolescents in the ICD–10 or the DSM–IV–TR.

REFERENCES

● REVIEWS ●

Benjamin S & Eminson D (1992) **Abnormal illness behaviour: childhood experiences and long-term consequences**. *International Review of Psychiatry*, **4**, 55–70.

Fritz G K, Fritsch S & Hagino O (1997) **Somatoform disorders in children and adolescents: a review of the past 10 years**. *Journal of the American Academy of Child and Adolescent Psychiatry*, **36**, 1329–1338.

Garralda M E (1999) **Practitioner review: assessment and management of somatisation in childhood and adolescence: a practical perspective**. *Journal of Psychology and Psychiatry*, **40**, 1159–1167.

Wright B, Partridge I & Williams C (2000) **Management of chronic fatigue syndrome in children**. *Advances in Psychiatric Treatment*, **6**, 145–152.

● CLINICAL GUIDELINES ●

None identified.

● CLASSIC PAPERS ●

Campo J V & Fritsch S (1994) **Somatization in children and adolescents**. *Journal of the American Academy of Child and Adolescent Psychiatry*, **33**, 1223–1235.

Sanders M R, Shepherd R W, Cleghorn G, *et al* (1994) **The treatment of recurrent abdominal pain in children: a controlled comparison of cognitive–behavioral family intervention and standard pediatric care**. *Journal of Consulting Clinical Psychology*, **62**, 515–529.

Taylor D C (1982) **The components of sickness: disease, illnesses and predicaments**. In *One Child* (eds J Apley & C Ounsted), pp. 1–13. London: Spastics International Medical Publications.

---

100 Mrazek D A (1994) Psychiatric aspects of somatic disease and disorders. In *Child and Adolescent Psychiatry: Modern Approaches* (eds M Rutter, E Taylor & L Hersov). 3rd edn. Oxford: Blackwell Scientific Publications.

● CUTTING EDGE PAPERS ●

Egger H L, Costello E J, Erkanli A, *et al* (1999) **Somatic complaints and psychopathology in children and adolescents: stock aches, musculo-skeletal pains and headaches**. *Journal of the American Academy of Child and Adolescent Psychiatry*, **38**, 852–860.

Hotopf M, Carr S, Mayou R, *et al* (1998) **Why do children have chronic abdominal pain, and what happens to then when they grow up? Population based cohort study.** *British Medical Journal*, **316**, 1196–1200.

Rangel L, Garralda M E, Levin M, *et al* (2000) **Personality in adolescents with chronic fatigue syndrome.** *European Child & Adolescent Psychiatry*, **9**, 39–45.

● FURTHER READING ●

Garralda E (1999) *Chronic Fatigue Syndrome: Helping Children and Adolescents*. Occasional Paper No. 16. London: Association for Child Psychology and Psychiatry.

Reid S, Chalder T, Cleare A, *et al* (2000) **Chronic fatigue syndrome.** *British Medical Journal*, **320**, 292–296.

PAEDIATRIC LIAISON: dying child

INTRODUCTION

Children and adolescents with life-threatening illnesses have a higher risk of developing psychiatric disorders. The need to undergo various forms of interventions, which may be painful, can lead to anxiety, depression and post-traumatic stress disorder.[101] It is important that mental health problems in this population are identified early so that adequate support can be given to them.

It is estimated that children with a chronic illness have double the risk of developing psychological problems compared with children without chronic illness.[102]

MANAGEMENT OF THE DYING CHILD

It is important that the medical and the psychiatric team work together to help the child and family deal to with the illness. Support for parents also becomes important to deal with the loss of their child. The time leading up to death is crucial to the functioning of the family and should be managed appropriately.[103]

It is also important for psychiatrists and psychologists to advise medical staff on some issues so that specific symptoms can be prevented and managed, for example needle phobia, anticipatory nausea anxiety (including death anxiety) and depression in children with a terminal illness.[104]

REFERENCES

● REVIEWS ●

Dyregrov A (1994) **Childhood bereavement consequences and therapeutic approaches**. *Association for Child Psychology and Psychiatry Review Newsletter*, **16**, July, 173–183.

Harrington R & Harrison L (1999) **Unproven assumptions about the impact of bereavement on children**. *Journal of the Royal Society of Medicine*, **92**, 230–233.

Stambrook M & Parker K C H (1987) **The development of the concept of death in childhood: a review of the literature**. *Merrill Palmer Quarterly*, **33**, 133–157.

● CLASSIC PAPERS ●

Bowlby J (1979) ***The Making and Breaking of Affectional Bonds***. London: Tavistock.

101 Black D, Cottrell D, Kaplan T, *et al* (1993) Liaison child and adolescent psychiatry. In *Seminars in Child and Adolescent Psychiatry* (eds D Black & D Cottrell), pp 249–275. London: Gaskell.
102 Mrazek D A (1994) Psychiatric aspects of somatic disease and disorders. In *Child and Adolescent Psychiatry: Modern Approaches* (eds M Rutter, E Taylor & L Hersov). 3rd edn. Oxford: Blackwell Scientific Publications.
103 Black D (1994) Psychological reactions to life-threatening and terminal illness bereavement. In *Child and Adolescent Psychiatry: Modern Approaches* (eds M Rutter, E Taylor & L Hersov). 3rd edn. Oxford: Blackwell Scientific Publications.
104 As above.

Kane B (1967) **Children's concepts of death**. *Journal of Genetic Psychiatry*, **17**, 593–597.

● GENERAL READING ●

Black D (1978) **The bereaved child**. *Journal of Child Psychology and Psychiatry*, **19**, 287–292.

Dyregrov A (1991) *Grief in Children. A Handbook for Adults*. London: Jessica Kingsley.

Earnshaw-Smith E (1982) **Emotional pain in dying patients and their families**. *Nursing Times*, **78**, 1865–1867.

Pettle S A & Britten C M (1995) **Talking with children about death and dying**. *Child Care, Health and Development*, **21**, 395–404.

● DEATH IN THE FAMILY ●

Ackworth A & Bruggen P (1985) **Family therapy when one member is on the death bed**. *Journal of Family Therapy*, **7**, 379–385.

Bisson J L & Cullum M (1994) **Group therapy for bereaved children**. *Association of Child Psychology and Psychiatry Review Newsletter*, **16**, 130–139.

Krasner S & Beinart H (1989) **The Monday Group: a brief intervention with the siblings of infants who died from SIDS**. *Association of Child Psychology and Psychiatry Newsletter*, **11**, 11–17.

Masterman S H & Reams R (1988) **Support groups for bereaved pre-school and school age children**. *American Journal of Orthopsychiatry*, **58**, 562–570.

Smith S & Pennells M (1991) **Bereaved children and adolescents**. In *Groupwork with Children and Adolescents: A Handbook* (ed. K Dwivedi), pp. 195–208. London: Jessica Kingsley.

● ON MORE UNUSUAL SITUATIONS ●

Harris-Hendricks J, Black D & Kaplan T (1993) *When Father Kills Mother: Guiding Children through Trauma and Grief*. London: Routledge.

Pettle S (1998) **Thinking about the future when death is inevitable: consultations in terminal care**. *Clinical Child Psychology and Psychiatry*, **3**, 131–139.

Udwin O (1993) **Children's reactions to trauma**. *Journal of Child Psychology and Psychiatry*, **34**, 115–127.

Young J (1991) **"Does mummy not want to see me?" Preparing a Three year old for the death of her mother**. In *Death, Dying and Society* (ed. C Newnes), pp. 386–397. Hove and London: Lawrence Erlbaum Associates. (First published as a special issue of *Changes: An International Journal of Psychology and Psychotherapy*, December 1990.)

Yule W & Gold A (1993) *Wise Before the Event. Coping with Crises in Schools*. London: Calouste Gulbenkian Foundation.

PERVASIVE DEVELOPMENTAL DISORDERS: Asperger's syndrome

Pervasive developmental disorders are severe distortions in basic psychological functions that are considered normal for various stages of development. It is estimated that in Great Britain 0.5% of boys and 0.1% of girls suffer from pervasive developmental disorders.[105]

The types of pervasive developmental disorders discussed in these two sections are Asperger's syndrome and autism.

INTRODUCTION

Children suffering from Asperger's syndrome have similar patterns of impairment as in autism (i.e. impairment in social interactions) except they have an average level of intelligence and no language delay. These children suffer from impaired social understanding, restrictive interests, and pragmatic difficulties.[106]

Asperger's syndrome is reported to be more likely to occur in males.[107] A study of children in England suggests that Asperger's syndrome occurs in 0.02–0.08% of children.[108]

DIAGNOSIS AND AETIOLOGY

The diagnosis of Asperger's syndrome is made on the basis of the presence of deficiencies in reciprocal social interactions, restrictive and repetitive behaviour and interests without any significant cognitive or language delay.[109]

In ICD–10, Asperger's syndrome falls in the subcategory of pervasive developmental disorders in the section on the disorders of psychological development. A diagnosis is made primarily on the basis of the child's behaviour and is much the same as the DSM–IV–TR criteria. The main symptoms include:

❍ severe impairment in social interaction;

❍ restricted behaviour, interests, activities; and

❍ no significant delay in language acquisition or cognitive development.

105 Meltzer H, Gatward R, Goodman R, *et al* (2000) *The Mental Health of Children and Adolescents in Great Britain*. London: The Stationery Office.

106 Le Couteur A (1993) **Clinical syndromes in early childhood**. In *Seminars in Child and Adolescent Psychiatry* (eds D Black & D Cottrell), pp. 95–123. London: Gaskell.
   Lord C & Rutter M (1994) **Autism and pervasive developmental disorders**. In *Child and Adolescent Psychiatry: Modern Approaches* (eds M Rutter, E Taylor & L Hersov). 3rd edn. Oxford: Blackwell Scientific Publications.

107 Wing & Gould (1979); Gillberg & Gillberg (1989) cited in Le Couteur A (1993) **Clinical syndromes in early childhood**. In *Seminars in Child and Adolescent Psychiatry* (eds D Black & D Cottrell), pp. 95–123. London: Gaskell.

108 Kurtz Z, Thornes R & Wolkind S (1996) *Services for the Mental Health of Children and Young People in England: Assessment of Needs and Unmet Needs*. London: South West Thames Regional Health Authority.

109 World Health Organization (1992) *The ICD–10 Classification of Mental and Behavioural Disorders: Clinical Descriptions and Diagnostic Guidelines*. Geneva: WHO.

by Dr Anne Gilchrist

What developments have there been in the management of Asperger's syndrome in the past 2–5 years ?

The concept of autistic spectrum disorders is increasingly used in clinical practice – sub-categorisations are of less interest.

Current research has tended to focus on a genetic basis for autistic spectrum disorders. Family studies have been shown to support the 'spectrum' concept.

The current management approaches of autistic spectrum disorders are primarily educational and social. Comorbid conditions can include ADHD and emotional and conduct disorders and may require separate treatment.

What are the key messages from new research that are not being widely used?

Children and adolescents can have severe communication handicaps despite superficially normal speech (that is, normal vocabulary and grammar).

Adequate performance in clinic test situations may be accompanied by lack of ability in real life situations. That is, information and observations outside the clinic setting are essential for diagnosis and management planning. No pattern of neuro-psychological results can itself be diagnostic of Asperger's syndrome.

REFERENCES

● SYSTEMATIC REVIEWS AND META-ANALYSES ●

Myhr G (1998) **Autism and other pervasive developmental disorders: exploring the dimensional view**. *Canadian Journal of Psychiatry*, **43**, 589–595.

Szatmari P (1992) **The validity of autistic spectrum disorders: a literature review**. *Journal of Autism and Developmental Disorders*, **22**, 583–600.

Tanguay P (2000) **Pervasive developmental disorders: A 10 year review**. *Journal of the American Academy of Child and Adolescent Psychiatry*, **39**, 1079–1095.

● PRACTICE PARAMETERS ●

American Academy of Child and Adolescent Psychiatry (1999) **Practice parameters for the assessment of treatment of children, adolescents, and adults with autism and other pervasive developmental disorders**. *Journal of the American Academy of Child and Adolescent Psychiatry*, **38** (suppl.), 32S–54S.

● REVIEWS ●

Filipek P A, Accardo P J & Baranek G T, *et al* (1999) **The screening and diagnosis of autistic spectrum disorders**. *Journal of Autism and Developmental Disorders*, **29**, 439–484.

Howlin P (2000) **Assessment instruments for Asperger's syndrome**. *Child Psychology and Psychiatry Review*, **5**, 120–128.

Volkmar F R (1998) **Categorical approaches to the diagnosis of autism: An overview of DSM–IV and ICD–10**. *Autism*, **2**, 45–59.

● CLASSIC PAPERS ●

Asperger H (1944) **Autistic psychopathy in childhood**. In *Autism and Asperger's syndrome* (translated and annotated by U Frith), pp. 93–121. New York: Cambridge University Press.

Bishop D (1989) **Autism, Asperger's syndrome and semantic-pragmatic disorder: where are the boundaries?** *British Journal of Disorders of Communication*, **24**, 107–121.

Wing L (1981) **Asperger's Syndrome: a clinical account**. *Psychological Medicine*, **11**, 115–129.

Wolff S (1991) **'Schizoid' personality in childhood and adult life – 1: The vagaries of diagnostic labelling**. *British Journal of Psychiatry*, **159**, 615–620.

Wolff S, Townshend R, McGuire R J, *et al* (1991) **'Schizoid' personality in childhood and adult life – II: Adult adjustment and the continuity with schizotypal personality disorder**. *British Journal of Psychiatry*, **159**, 620–629.

● CUTTING EDGE PAPERS ●

Klin A (2000) **Attributing social meaning to ambiguous visual stimuli in higher-functioning autism and Asperger syndrome**. *Journal of Child Psychology and Psychiatry*, **41**, 831–846.

Miller J N & Ozonoff S (2000) **The external validity of Asperger disorder: Lack of evidence from the domain of neuropsychology**. *Journal of Abnormal Psychology*, **109**, 227–238.

Robertson J M, Tanguay P, L'Ecuyer S, *et al* (1999) **Domains of social communication handicap in autistic spectrum disorder**. *Journal of the American Academy of Child and Adolescent Psychiatry*, **38**, 738–745.

Schultz R T, Gauthier I, Klin A, *et al* (2000) **Abnormal ventral temporal cortical activity during face discrimination among individuals with autism and Asperger syndrome**. *Archives of General Psychiatry*, **57**, 344–346.

Szatmari P, MacLean J E & Jones M B (2000) **The familial aggregation of the lesser variant in biological and nonbiological relatives of PDD probands: A family history study**. *Journal of Child Psychology and Psychiatry*, **41**, 831–846.

● BOOKS ●

Attwood T (1998) *Asperger's Syndrome – A Guide for Parents and Professionals*. London: Jessica Kingsley.

Happe F (1994) *Autism: An Introduction to Psychological Theory*. London: University College London Press.

Klin A & Volkmar F R (1997) **Asperger syndrome**. In *Handbook of Autism and Pervasive Developmental Disorders* (eds D J Cohen & F R Volkmar), pp. 94–122. New York: Wiley and Sons.

On-line Asperger Syndrome Information and Support http://udel.edu/bkirby/asperger/

Cochrane Controlled Trials Register

14 hits (keywords: pervasive developmental disorder*)
0 hits (keywords: aspergers syndrome)
4 hits (keywords: asperger syndrome)

Cochrane Developmental, Psychosocial and Learning Problems Group
Contacts: Dr Jane Dennis, Review Group Coordinator, Bristol University, UK.
j.dennis@bristol.ac.uk

INTRODUCTION

Autism (otherwise known as infantile autism, childhood autism or Kanner's autism) is a neurodevelopmental disorder characterised by cognitive and social difficulties and is the prototypical pervasive developmental disorder.

The hallmarks of autism are impairments in reciprocal social interaction and communication and the presence of repetitive or stereotyped interests and activities. This means that a child with autism may be unable to use language appropriately to participate in conversation and may also lack emotional expression in his or her use of language. A child with autism is unlikely to show spontaneous affection, may prefer to be on his or her own and may not show normal separation anxiety. Essentially, these children find it difficult to understand and respond to simple social and emotional cues.[110] The manifestation of autism varies according to the developmental level and age of the child.[111]

The prevalence rates of autism vary. From studies conducted since 1987, it is estimated that the prevalence of autism is 7.5 cases per 10 000 individuals, with an additional 12.25 cases per 10 000 individuals having atypical autism or pervasive developmental disorder. Thus, the overall prevalence of pervasive developmental disorder is estimated at 20 cases per 10 000 individuals.[112]

DIAGNOSIS AND AETIOLOGY

According to the ICD-10, childhood autism can only be diagnosed if behavioural abnormalities manifest before the age of three years. Symptoms must include abnormal social interactions, communication and restricted and/or repetitive behaviour. Atypical autism can be diagnosed if the age of onset criteria or abnormal functioning in the three areas are not all met.

The DSM-IV-TR uses the same criteria for the diagnosis of autism as the ICD-10 but adds that for a diagnosis of autism to be made the disturbance observed should not be better accounted for by Rett's disorder or childhood disintegrative disorder.

The aetiology of autism is uncertain. In a small proportion of cases, autism is associated with recognised medical disorders (chromosomal abnormalities, fragile X and tuberous sclerosis). Twin and family studies suggest that a complex genetic predisposition is relevant in the majority of individuals.

CRITICAL QUESTIONS

by Dr Anthony Bailey

What developments have there been in the management of autism in the past 2–5 years?

A diagnostic assessment should include a comprehensive developmental history as well as observation of the child. Several diagnostic interviews are available and the Autism Diagnostic Observation Schedule (ADOS) provides a semi-structured

110 Le Couteur A (1993) Clinical syndromes in early childhood. In *Seminars in Child and Adolescent Psychiatry* (eds D Black & D Cottrell), pp. 95–123. London: Gaskell.
111 World Health Organization (1992) *The ICD-10 Classification of Mental and Behavioural Disorders: Clinical Descriptions and Diagnostic Guidelines*. Geneva: WHO.
112 Fombonne E (1999) The epidemiology of autism: a review. *Psychological Medicine*, 29, 769–786.

observational framework. Children with autism and other pervasive developmental disorders are often at their best in structured one-to-one interactions with adults, and nursery or school-based observation of interactions with peers is often useful when the diagnosis is uncertain. Although the rate of causal medical conditions is relatively low, all affected children should have a full physical examination, karyotyping and molecular genetic testing for fragile X as a matter of course. There has recently been a particular focus on identifying autism susceptibility loci, and future success is likely to be relevant to clinical practice. Recent post-mortem studies suggest relatively widespread developmental abnormalities, and macrocephaly is, by itself, not an indication for neuroimaging.

What are the key messages from new research that are not being widely used?

Parents of newly diagnosed children should be counselled about the elevated risk of having further affected children.

Educational provision should be tailored to the individual. Children with social difficulties who are educated in mainstream settings are at risk from bullying.

Optimal care involves careful management of the transition to adult services.

REFERENCES

● SYSTEMATIC REVIEWS AND META-ANALYSES ●

Best L & Milne R (1997) *Auditory Integration Training in Autism*. Southampton: Wessex Institute for Health Research and Development. DEC Report no 66. (Reviewed in *The Cochrane Library*.)

Law J, Boyle J, Harris F, *et al* (1998) **Screening for speech and language delay: A systematic review of the literature**. *Health Technology Assessment*, **2**, 1–184.

Yirmiya N, Erel O, Shaked M, *et al* (1998) **Meta-analyses comparing theory of mind abilities of individuals with autism, individuals with mental retardation, and normally developing individuals**. *Psychological Bulletin*, **124**, 283–307.

● PRACTICE PARAMETERS ●

Filipek P A, Accardo P J, Ashwal S, *et al* (2000) **Practice parameter: Screening and diagnosis of autism: Report of the Quality Standards Subcommittee of the American Academy of Neurology and the Child Neurology Society**. *Neurology*, **55**, 468–479.

Volkmar F, Cook E H J, Pomeroy J, *et al* (1999) **Practice parameters for the assessment and treatment of children, adolescents, and adults with autism and other pervasive developmental disorders**. American Academy of Child and Adolescent Psychiatry Working Group on Quality Issues. *Journal of the American Academy of Child and Adolescent Psychiatry*, **38**, 32S–54S.

● CLINICAL GUIDELINES ●

Curry C J, Stevenson R E, Aughton D, *et al* (1997) **Evaluation of mental retardation: Recommendations of a consensus conference: American College of Medical Genetics**. *American Journal of Medical Genetics*, **72**, 468–477.

Freeman B J (1997) **Guidelines for evaluating intervention programs for children with autism**. *Journal of Autism and Developmental Disorders*, **27**, 641–651.

● REVIEWS ●

Bailey A, Phillips W & Rutter M (1996) **Autism: towards an integration of clinical, genetic, neuropsychological and neurobiological perspectives**. *Journal of Child Psychology and Psychiatry and Allied Disciplines*, **37**, 89–126.

Flavell J H (1999) **Cognitive development: Children's knowledge about the mind**. *Annual Review of Psychology*, **50**, 21–45.

Fombonne E (1999) **The epidemiology of autism: a review**. *Psychological Medicine*, **29**, 769–786.

Happe F & Frith U (1996) **The neuropsychology of autism**. *Brain*, **119**, 1377–1400.

Howlin P (1997) **Prognosis in autism: do specialist treatments affect long-term outcome?** *European Child and Adolescent Psychiatry*, **6**, 55–72.

—— (1998) **Practitioner review: Psychological and educational treatments for autism**. *Journal of Child Psychology and Psychiatry and Allied Disciplines*, **39**, 307–322.

Pennington B & Ozonoff S (1996) **Executive functions and developmental psychopathology**. *Journal of Child Psychology and Psychiatry*, **37**, 51–87.

Towbin K E (1997) **Autism and Asperger's syndrome**. *Current Opinion in Pediatrics*, **9**, 361–366.

Turner M (1999) **Annotation: Repetitive behaviour in autism: a review of psychological research**. *Journal of Child Psychology and Psychiatry*, **40**, 839–849.

Vostanis P, Smith B, Chung M C, *et al* (1994) **Early detection of childhood autism: a review of screening instructions and rating scales**. *Child: Care, Health and Development*, **20**, 165–177.

Wetherby A M & Prizant B M (1999) **Enhancing language and communication development in autism: Assessment and intervention guidelines**. In *Autism: Identification, Education, and Treatment* (ed. D B Zager), pp. 141–174. 2nd edn. Mahwah, NJ: Lawrence Erlbaum Associates.

● CLASSIC PAPERS ●

Bolton P, MacDonald H, Pickles A, *et al* (1994) **A case control family history study of autism**. *Journal of Child Psychology and Psychiatry*, **35**, 887–900.

Kanner L (1943) **Autistic disturbances of affective contact**. *Nervous Child*, **2**, 217–250.

Rutter M (1999) **The Emanuel Miller Memorial Lecture 1998. Autism: Two-way interplay between research and clinical work**. *Journal of Child Psychology and Psychiatry and Allied Disciplines*, **40**, 169–188.

Smalley S (1998) **Autism and tuberous sclerosis**. *Journal of Autism and Developmental Disorders*, **28** (special issue), 407–414.

● CUTTING EDGE PAPERS ●

Bailey A, Luthert P, Harding B, *et al* (1998) **A clinicopathological study of autism**. *Brain*, **121**, 889–905.

Gilchrist A, Green J, Cox A, *et al* (2001) **Development and current functioning in adolescents with Asperger syndrome: A comparative study**. *Journal of Child Psychology and Psychiatry and Allied Disciplines*, **42**, 227–240.

Minshew N J, Luna B & Sweeney J A (1999) **Oculomotor evidence for neocortical systems but not cerebellar dysfunction in autism.** *Neurology*, **52**, 917–922.

Nicoll A, Elliman D & Ross E (1998) **MMR vaccination and autism 1998**. *British Medical Journal*, **316**, 715–716.

Piven J, Arndt S, Bailey J, *et al* (1996) **Regional brain enlargement in autism: a magnetic imaging study**. *Journal of the American Academy of Child and Adolescent Psychiatry*, **35**, 530–536.

Woodhouse W, Bailey A, Bolton P, *et al* (1996) **Head circumference and pervasive developmental disorder**. *Journal of Child Psychology and Psychiatry*, **37**, 665–671.

● GENETIC BASIS OF AUTISM ●

Bailey A, Le Couteur A, Gottesman I, *et al* (1995) **Autism as a strongly genetic disorder: evidence from a British twin study**. *Psychological Medicine*, **2**, 63–77.

Cook E H, Lindgren V, Leventhal B L, *et al* (1997) **Autism or atypical autism in maternally but not paternally derived proximal 15q duplication**. *American Journal of Human Genetics*, **60**, 928–934.

Feinstein C & Reiss A L (1998) **Autism: the point of view from fragile X studies.** *Journal of Autism and Developmental Disorders*, **28** (special issue), 393–405.

International Molecular Genetics Study of Autism Consortium (IMGSAC) (2001) **Further characterization of the autism susceptibility locus AUTS1 on chromosome 7q**. *Human Molecular Genetics*, **10**, 973–982.

Lamb J A, Moore J, Bailey A, *et al* (2000) **Autism: recent molecular genetic advances**. *Human Molecular Genetics*, **9**, 861–868.

Pickles A, Bolton P, MacDonald H, *et al* (1995) **Latent class analysis of recurrence risks for complex phenotypes with selection and measurement error: a twin and family history study of autism**. *American Journal of Human Genetics*, **57**, 717–726.

Simonoff E (1998) **Genetic counselling in autism and pervasive developmental disorders**. *Journal of Autism and Developmental Disorders*, **28** (special issue), 447–456.

Szatmari P, Jones M B, Zwaigenbaum L, *et al* (1998) **Genetics of autism: Overview and new directions**. *Journal of Autism and Developmental Disorders*, **28**, 351–368.

● OTHER PAPERS ●

Lord C, Risi S, Lambrecht L, *et al* (2000) **The autism diagnostic observation schedule-generic: A standard measure of social and communication deficits associated with the spectrum of autism**. *Journal of Autism and Developmental Disorders*, **30**, 205–223.

Potenza M N, Holmes J P, Kanes S J, *et al* (1999) **Olanzapine treatment of children, adolescents, and adults with pervasive developmental disorders: an open label pilot study**. *Journal of Clinical Psychopharmacology*, **19**, 37–44.

● BOOKS ●

Cohen D J & Folkmar F R (1997) *Handbook of Autism and Pervasive Developmental Disorders* (2nd edn). New York: John Wiley and Sons.

Howlin P (1998) *Children with Autism and Asperger Syndrome: A Guide for Practitioners and Carers*. Chichester: John Wiley and Sons.

Volkmar F R (1998) *Autism and Pervasive Developmental Disorders*. Cambridge: Cambridge University Press.

● USEFUL WEBSITES ●

Autism Society of America (ASA) http://www.autism-society.org

National Autistic Society (UK) http://www.oneworld.org/autism_uk

Center for the Study of Autism http://www.autism.org

Cochrane Controlled Trials Register
156 hits (keywords: autism)
178 hits (keyword: autistic)

Cochrane Developmental, Psychosocial and Learning Problems Group
Contact: Dr Jane Dennis, Bristol, UK. J.Dennis@bristol.ac.uk

POST-TRAUMATIC STRESS DISORDER

INTRODUCTION

The symptoms of post-traumatic stress disorder (PTSD) can vary according to the nature of the trauma. The most common symptoms are heightened anxiety, recurrent intrusive thoughts, images, memories or flashbacks, sleep disturbances, avoidance of similar situations as the original trauma, repetitive play, drawings of the event and the inability to concentrate. It is not uncommon for children to show various forms of regressive and antisocial behaviour.[113]

PTSD is estimated to occur in 0.2% of children in Great Britain.[114]

DIAGNOSIS AND AETIOLOGY

It is thought that children previously exposed to traumatic events are more prone to develop PTSD after a further significant individual stressor than children who have not experienced other traumas.[115] The effects of PTSD can be compounded by the experience of multiple or ongoing traumas, such as in the case of physical and sexual abuse.

There is no specific category for PTSD for children, but a general diagnostic category for adults and children in both the DSM–IV–TR and the ICD–10. For a diagnosis to be made, it must be thought that the symptoms are a direct result of the exceptionally stressful life event (exceptionally threatening or catastrophic in nature) or continued trauma.[116] The symptoms must include: (1) intense fear or helplessness during the traumatic event; (2) re-experiencing of the event; (3) avoidance of stimuli associated with the trauma and numbing of responses; and (4) persistent increased arousal. The onset of the symptoms must occur within six months of the event.[117]

CRITICAL QUESTIONS

by Dr Martin Newman

What developments have there been in the management of post-traumatic stress disorder in the past 2–5 years?

There is increasing evidence for the cross-cultural validity of PTSD.

CBT has become increasingly recognised as useful in the treatment of PTSD.

113 Berelowitz M & Nelki J (1993) **Clinical syndromes in middle childhood**. In *Seminars in Child and Adolescent Psychiatry* (eds D Black & D Cottrell), pp. 124–153. London: Gaskell.

114 Meltzer H & Gatward R (2000) *The Mental Health of Children and Adolescents in Great Britain*. London: The Stationery Office.

115 Yule W (1994) **Posttraumatic stress disorders**. In *Child and Adolescent Psychiatry: Modern Approaches* (eds M Rutter, E Taylor & L Hersov). 3rd edn. Oxford: Blackwell Scientific Publications.

116 World Health Organization (1992) *The ICD–10 Classification of Mental and Behavioural Disorders: Clinical Descriptions and Diagnostic Guidelines*. Geneva: WHO.

117 American Psychiatric Association (2000) *Diagnostic and Statistical Manual of Mental Disorders*. 4th edn (DSM–IV–TR). Washington DC: APA.

What are the key messages from new research that are not being widely used?

Psychological debriefing is ineffective and may have adverse long-term effects. It is not a necessary intervention for those who have experienced traumatic events.

REFERENCES

● CLINICAL EVIDENCE ●

Bisson J (2000) **Post-traumatic stress disorder**. In *Clinical Evidence. A Compendium of the Best Available Evidence for Effective Health Care*, Issue 4, pp. 552–557. London: BMJ Publishing Group.

● SYSTEMATIC REVIEWS AND META-ANALYSES ●

Everly G S, Boyle S H & Lating J M (1999) **The effectiveness of psychological debriefing with vicarious trauma: A meta-analysis**. *Stress Medicine*, **15**, 229–233.

Stein D J, Zungu-Dirwayi N, Van der Linden G, *et al* (2001) **Pharmacotherapy for post traumatic stress disorder**. Cochrane Review. In *The Cochrane Library*, Issue 1. Oxford: Update Software.

Wessely S, Rose S & Bisson J (1997) **Brief psychological interventions ('debriefing') for treating trauma-related symptoms and preventing post traumatic stress disorder**. Cochrane Review. In *The Cochrane Library*, Issue 1. Oxford: Update Software. (For ages 16 years and onward.)

● PRACTICE PARAMETERS ●

American Academy of Child and Adolescent Psychiatry (1998) **Practice parameters for the assessment and treatment of children and adolescents with post-traumatic stress disorder**. *Journal of the American Academy of Child and Adolescent Psychiatry*, **37** (suppl.), 4S–26S.

● CLINICAL GUIDELINES ●

Foa E B, Davidson J R T & Frances A (eds) (1999) The expert consensus guideline series. **Treatment of post traumatic stress disorder. The expert consensus panels for PTSD**. *Journal of Clinical Psychiatry*, **60** (suppl. 16), 3–76.

● REVIEWS ●

Perrin S, Smith P & Yule W (2000) **Practitioner review: The assessment and treatment of post traumatic stress disorder in children and adolescents**. *Journal of Child Psychology and Psychiatry*, **41**, 277–289.

Pfefferbaum B (1998) **Post traumatic stress disorder in children: a review of the past 10 years**. *Journal of the American Academy of Child and Adolescent Psychiatry*, **36**, 1503–1511.

Udwin O (1993) **Children's reactions to traumatic events**. *Journal of Child Psychology and Psychiatry*, **34**, 115–127.

● CLASSIC PAPERS ●

Horowitz M, Wilner N & Alvariz W (1979) **Impact of event scale: a measure of subjective stress**. *Psychosomatic Medicine*, **41**, 209–218.

Scheeringa M S, Zeanah C H, Drell M J, *et al* (1995) **Two approaches to diagnosing post-traumatic stress disorder in infancy and early childhood**. *Journal of the American Academy of Child and Adolescent Psychiatry*, **34**, 191–200.

● CUTTING EDGE PAPERS ●

Cahill S P, Carrigan M H & Frieh B C (1999) **Does EMDR work? And if so, why? A critical review of controlled outcome and dismantling research**. *Journal of Anxiety Disorders*, **13**, 5–33.

Simon R I (1999) **Chronic post traumatic stress disorder: A review and checklist of factors influencing prognosis**. *Harvard Review of Psychiatry*, **6**, 304–312.

● BOOKS ●

Black D, Harris-Hendriks J & Kaplan T (1993) *When Father Kills Mother: Guiding Children through Trauma and Grief*. London: Routledge.

● FURTHER READING ●

Cicchetti D & Toth S L (1997) *Developmental Perspectives on Trauma: Theory, Research, and Intervention. Rochester Symposium on Developmental Psychopathology*. Vol. 8. Rochester, NY: University of Rochester Press.

Davidson J R & Connor K M (1999) **Management of post traumatic stress disorder: Diagnostic and therapeutic issues**. *Journal of Clinical Psychiatry*, **60** (suppl.), 33–38.

Joseph S, Williams R & Yule W (1997) *Understanding Post-Traumatic Stress: A Psychosocial Perspective on PTSD and Treatment*. Chichester: Wiley.

● USEFUL WEBSITES ●

Post Traumatic Stress Disorder Bibliography   http://www.sover.net/~schwcof/ptsd.html

---

Cochrane Controlled Trials Register
24 hits (keywords: post traumatic stress AND child*)
34 hits (keywords: post traumatic stress AND adolescen*)

Cochrane Depression, Anxiety and Neurosis Group
Contact: Dr Natalie Khin, Review Group Coordinator, New Zealand.
n.khin@auckland.ac.nz

PSYCHOSIS: mania and bipolar affective disorder

INTRODUCTION

Bipolar affective disorder, otherwise known as manic-depressive illness, is a mood disorder characterised by severe mood swings that regress and reoccur.

Mania is characterised by elevated mood and an increase in the quantity and speed of both physical and mental activity.[118]

Bipolar affective disorders are more common after puberty than in childhood.[119] Figures suggest that bipolar disorder occurs in 0.2% of children in the 7–11-year age group and in 0.66% of adolescents.[120]

DIAGNOSIS AND AETIOLOGY

The ICD–10 details criteria for the diagnosis of manic episodes and bipolar affective disorders. Manic episodes are categorised into three degrees of severity of the disorder. These are:

○ hypomania (lesser degree of mania);

○ mania without psychotic symptoms; and

○ mania with psychotic symptoms (psychotic symptoms can include delusions of grandeur and identity, hallucinations, etc.).

The DSM–IV–TR does not categorise manic episodes in degrees of severity but includes diagnoses for manic episodes, mixed episodes and hypomanic episodes under the section on mood episodes.

According to the ICD–10, bipolar affective disorders can be categorised into one of eight categories that describe the current episode. The DSM–IV–TR uses similar categories to the ICD–10, although only six categories are used for diagnosis. The DSM–IV–TR also categorises bipolar disorders as bipolar I for the first episode of mania and bipolar II for individuals who have recurrent mood episodes.

Hyperactivity and distractibility are common symptoms of bipolar disorders in children and adolescents. However, older children (9–12 years of age) exhibit symptoms such as grandiose thoughts and paranoia, whereas younger children seem to show signs of irritability and emotional instability. It has also been suggested that younger children with bipolar disorders experience many brief cycles of a mixture of dysphoria and hypomania, whereas adolescents experience cycles with the extremes of depression and mania.[121]

118 World Health Organization (1992) *The ICD–10 Classification of Mental and Behavioural Disorders: Clinical Descriptions and Diagnostic Guidelines*. Geneva: WHO.

119 Berelowitz M & Nelki J (1993) Clinical syndromes in middle childhood. In *Seminars in Child and Adolescent Psychiatry* (eds D Black & D Cottrell), pp. 124–153. London: Gaskell.

120 Kurtz Z, Thornes R & Wolkind S (1996) *Services for the Mental Health of Children and Young People in England: Assessment of Needs and Unmet Needs*. London: South West Thames Regional Health Authority.

121 Harrington R (1994) Affective disorders. In *Child and Adolescent Psychiatry: Modern Approaches* (eds M Rutter E, Taylor & L Hersov). 3rd edn. Oxford: Blackwell Scientific Publications.

It is often difficult to distinguish between mania and bipolar affective disorders and schizophrenic type disorders.[122]

Genetic factors are said to have a role in the aetiology of bipolar disorders.[123]

CRITICAL QUESTIONS

by Dr Garry Wannan and Dr Paramala Santosh

What new developments have there been in the management of mania and bipolar affective disorders in the past 2–5 years?

Dr Garry Wannan   Relatively little research has been undertaken in the field of child and adolescent mania. Practice with children has largely been formed by adult research, in which a major development has been the use of new drugs in the treatment and prophylaxis of bipolar disorder. Lithium salts have been the mainstay of treatment for more than 50 years, but now an increasing number of atypical antipsychotics (including olanzapine and risperidone) and anticonvulsants (carbamazepine initially but joined by others as valproate and lamotrigine) are commonly used. Many of these drugs offer side-effect profiles considerably better than lithium, but their prophylactic efficacy has not yet been established in trials among adults. Owing to continuing issues of licensing and relatively small population numbers, drug trials in young people are unlikely to be performed in the near future.

Dr Paramala Santosh   Recently there has been a resurfacing of the debate regarding the possible existence of pre-pubertal bipolar illness. Proponents of a childhood bipolar diagnosis argue that there is an early-onset form of bipolar illness that is highly comorbid and characterised by simultaneous irritability and depression. Others have suggested that childhood manic symptoms are more likely a non-specific indicator of risk, or may be the result of symptom overlap with various forms of childhood pathology. Rapid cycling affective disorder is reported to be a very common subtype seen in this age group. The major difficulties that complicate the diagnosis of paediatric mania include its overlap with ADHD, aggression, conduct disorder, and substance use disorders, and its atypical response (by adult standards) to treatment. Research does not implicate stimulants in the aetiology of bipolar disorder in children with ADHD.

Neuroimaging using proton magnetic resonance spectroscopy in children with bipolar affective disorder has recently shown abnormalities in both frontal lobes and basal ganglia and raises possibilities of illness markers in the future.

What are the key messages from new research that are not being widely used?

Dr Garry Wannan and Dr Paramala Santosh   Clinicians in child and adolescent mental health are faced with the typical problem of extrapolating adult studies on drugs licensed for use in adults when considering medical treatment for a young person with bipolar disorder.

---

122 Werry J S & Taylor E (1994) *Schizophrenic and allied disorders. In Child and Adolescent Psychiatry: Modern Approaches* (eds M Rutter, E Taylor & L Hersov). 3rd edn. Oxford: Blackwell Scientific Publications.
123 Harrington R (1994) **Affective disorders**. In *Child and Adolescent Psychiatry: Modern Approaches* (eds M Rutter, E Taylor & L Hersov). 3rd edn. Oxford: Blackwell Scientific Publications.

Recent studies have shown very high rates of switching to mania in pre-pubertal major depressive disorder, especially when associated with psychotic features. Increasingly, it is becoming necessary to rule out bipolar illness in children who present with 'difficult to treat' neurodevelopmental disorders.

Psychiatrists may not think in the first instance of a diagnosis of bipolar disorder, particularly if there are family and social factors that are causing a young person to be mentally ill. These difficulties may lead to a lack of readiness to prescribe medication in bipolar disorder. Psychiatrists should use a bio-psychosocial approach and view drug treatment, family, psychological and social interventions as part of their holistic approach to treatment. It is important to point out that that the limited evidence for the use of several anti-manic preparations in children is promising. Preliminary data, however, suggest that sodium valproate should be used as the first line of treatment in this population, and two or more mood stabilisers may become necessary to adequately control rapid cycling affective disorder subtype.

REFERENCES

● CLINICAL EVIDENCE ●

Bipolar disorder has been commissioned for future issues of *Clinical Evidence*.

● SYSTEMATIC REVIEWS AND META-ANALYSES ●

Botteron K N & Geller B (1995) **Pharmacologic treatment of childhood and adolescent mania**. *Child and Adolescent Psychiatric Clinics of North America*, **4**, 283–304.

Geller B & Luby J (1997) **Child and adolescent bipolar disorder: a review of the past 10 years**. *Journal of the American Academy of Child and Adolescent Psychiatry*, **36**, 1168–1176. (Erratum in **36**, 1642.)

Kutcher S & Robertson H A (1995) **Electroconvulsive therapy in treatment-resistant bipolar youth**. *Journal of Child and Adolescent Psychopharmacology*, **5**, 167–175.

Lapalme M, Hodgins S & LaRoche C (1997) **Children of parents with bipolar disorder: a metaanalysis of risk for mental disorders**. *Canadian Journal of Psychiatry*, **42**, 623–631.

Poolsup N, Li-Wan P A & de Oliveira I R (2000) **Systematic overview of lithium treatment in acute mania**. *Journal of Clinical Pharmacological Therapy*, **25**, 139–156.

Weller E B, Weller R A & Fristad M A (1995) **Bipolar disorder in children: misdiagnosis, underdiagnosis, and future directions**. *Journal of the American Academy of Child and Adolescent Psychiatry*, **34**, 709–714.

● PRACTICE PARAMETERS ●

American Academy of Child and Adolescent Psychiatry (1997) **Practice parameters for the assessment and treatment of children and adolescents with bipolar disorders**. *Journal of the American Academy of Child and Adolescent Psychiatry*, **36** (suppl.), 157S–173S.

● CLINICAL GUIDELINES ●

Frances A, Docherty J P & Kahn D A (eds) (1996) **The expert consensus guideline series: Treatment of bipolar disorder**. *Journal of Clinical Psychiatry*, **58** (suppl.).

Sachs G S, Printz D J, Kahn D A, *et al* (2000) **Expert consensus guideline series: Medication treatment of bipolar disorder**. *Postgraduate Medicine*, April (special number), 1–104.

● REVIEWS ●

Carlson G A & Meyer S E (2000) **Bipolar disorder in youth**. *Current Psychiatry Report*, **2**, 90–94.

Davanso P A & McCracken J T (2000) **Mood stabilizers in the treatment of juvenile bipolar disorder. Advances and controversies**. *Child and Adolescent Psychiatric Clinics of North America*, **9**, 159–182.

Geller B & Luby J (1997) **Child and adolescent bipolar disorder: a review of the past 10 years**. *Journal of the American Academy of Child and Adolescent Psychiatry*, **36**, 1168–1176.

James A C D & Javaloyes A M (2001) **The treatment of bipolar disorders in children and adolescents**. *Journal of Child Psychology and Psychiatry*, **42**, 439–449.

● CLASSIC PAPERS ●

Anthony E J & Scott P (1960) **Manic depressive psychosis in childhood**. *Journal of Child Psychology and Psychiatry*, **1**, 53–72.

Kreapelin E (1921) *Manic Depressive Insanity and Paranore*. Edinburgh: Churchill Livingstone.

Loranger A P W & Levine P M (1978) **Age of onset of bipolar affective illness**. *Archives of General Psychiatry*, **35**, 1345–1348.

● CUTTING EDGE PAPERS ●

Castillo M, Kwock L, Courvoise H, *et al* (2000) **Proton MR spectroscopy in children with bipolar affective disorder: preliminary observations**. *American Journal of Neuroradiology*, **21**, 832–838.

Chang K D & Ketter T A (2000) **Mood stabilizer augmentation with olanzapine in acutely manic children**. *Journal of Child and Adolescent Psychopharmacology*, **10**, 45–49.

Frazier J A, Meyer M C, Bierderman J, *et al* (1999) **Risperidone treatment for juvenile bipolar disorder: A retrospective chart review**. *Journal of the American Academy of Child and Adolescent Psychiatry*, **38**, 960–965.

Geller B, Cooper T B, Sun K, *et al* (1998) **Double-blind placebo-controlled study of lithium for adolescents with comorbid bipolar and substance dependency**. *Journal of the American Academy of Child and Adolescent Psychiatry*, **37**, 171–178.

Kowatch R A, Suppes T, Carmody T J, *et al* (2000) **Effect of lithium, divalproex sodium, and carbamazepine in children and adolescents with bipolar disorder**. *Journal of the American Academy of Child and Adolescent Psychiatry*, **39**, 713–720.

Remschmidt H (1998) **Bipolar disorders in children and adolescents**. *Current Opinion in Psychiatry*, **11**, 379–383.

Sigurdsson E, Fombonne E, Sayal K, *et al* (1999) **Neurodevelopmental antecedents of early-onset bipolar affective disorder**. *British Journal of Psychiatry*, **174**, 121–127.

● USEFUL WEBSITES ●

Mind http://www.mind.org.uk

Cochrane Controlled Trials Register
6 hits (keywords: mania AND child*)
34 hits (keywords: mania AND adoles*)
32 hits (keywords: bipolar disorder AND child*)
142 hits (keywords: bipolar disorder AND adolesc*)

Cochrane Depression, Anxiety and Neurosis Group
Contact: Dr Natalie Khin, Review Group Coordinator, New Zealand.
n.khin@auckland.ac.nz

PSYCHOSIS: schizophrenia

INTRODUCTION

Schizophrenia is characterised by abnormalities in thinking, perception and emotion.[124] It has been suggested that differences between childhood schizophrenia and adult schizophrenia are mostly developmental and quantitative.[125]

The onset of schizophrenia is usually between the ages of 15 and 35 years, but has more recently been recognised to occur in childhood.

DIAGNOSIS AND AETIOLOGY

Both the ICD–10 and DSM–IV–TR use the same diagnostic criteria for the diagnosis of schizophrenia for children and adolescents as for adults.

The ICD–10 diagnostic criteria focuses primarily on the conceptual basis of schizophrenia and the types of symptoms that arise. Thus, a diagnosis of schizophrenia using ICD–10 criteria would require a fair deal of clinical judgement. However, the DSM–IV–TR has very strict diagnostic criteria and very clear clinical guidelines.[126]

The positive symptoms of schizophrenia include: delusions, hallucinations, thought disorder, as well as excitement and paranoid tendencies. Negative symptoms usually involve a numbing or dulling of affect, apathy, lack of interest in socialising, and anhedonia.[127]

The developmental variations in child and adolescent schizophrenia include rather infrequent occurrences of poverty of thinking, incoherence and passivity. Delusions in children are also less complex and frequent than in adults. Care should be exercised in defining hallucinations in childhood, as children may find it difficult to describe their hallucinations.[128] The classic schizophrenic symptoms begin to appear in late adolescence and commonly include blunting of affect, social withdrawal and social as well as educational difficulties.[129]

It seems that a history of passivity, short attention span and poor emotional control behaviours precede an early onset of schizophrenia.[130]

CRITICAL QUESTIONS

by Professor Chris Hollis and Dr Paramala Santosh

What new developments have there been in the management of schizophrenia in the past 2–5 years?

Professor Chris Hollis   Longitudinal structural brain imaging studies have revealed two important findings:

124 World Health Organization (1992) *The ICD–10 Classification of Mental and Behavioural Disorders: Clinical Descriptions and Diagnostic Guidelines*. Geneva: WHO.

125 Werry J S & Taylor E (1994) **Schizophrenic and allied disorders**. In *Child and Adolescent Psychiatry: Modern Approaches* (eds M Rutter, E Taylor & L Hersov). 3rd edn. Oxford: Blackwell Scientific Publications.

126 As 124 above.

127 As 124 above.

128 As 124 above.

129 Scarth L (1993) **Clinical syndromes in adolescence**. In *Seminars in Child and Adolescent Psychiatry* (eds D Black & D Cottrell), pp. 154–182. London: Gaskell.

130 Smalley *et al* (1999) cited in Le Couteur A (1993) **Clinical syndromes in early childhood**. In *Seminars in Child and Adolescent Psychiatry* (eds D Black & D Cottrell), pp. 95–123. London: Gaskell.

1. There is evidence that typical antipsychotics can produce structural changes in the basal ganglia that are reversible after transfer to clozapine.[131]

2. There is evidence for progressive structural brain changes affecting the temporal and frontal lobes in the early phase of illness.[132]

Longitudinal follow-up of child and adolescent-onset psychoses has also shown that schizophrenia diagnosed using DSM–III–R/DSM–IV criteria has good diagnostic stability and predictive validity into adult life. Studies of prognostic indicators suggest that the presence at onset of negative symptoms and premorbid impairments predicts long-term disability.[133]

The most significant development in management has been the introduction of a wider range of atypical antipsychotics (e.g. olanzapine, quetiapine, ziprasidone, zotepine). These drugs have significantly reduced risk of producing extrapyramidal side-effects and tardive dyskinesia. There remains a lack of studies evaluating the benefits of newer antipsychotics in child and adolescent patients.

Dr Paramala Santosh   Clinicians have increasingly become interested in studying early-onset schizophrenia, and have tried to classify this disorder into pre-pubertal/childhood-onset schizophrenia and post-pubertal subtypes (with an arbitrary cut-off of 12 or 14 years of age at onset). Childhood-onset schizophrenia is a rare and severe form of the disorder that is clinically and neurobiologically continuous with the adult-onset disorder. Adolescence appears to play a role in increasing psychoses in children, especially boys, owing to a unique neurohormonal influences and differential brain development.

Current treatment strategies involve the use of atypical antipsychotics such as risperidone or olanzapine as the first-line treatment. On the basis of pharmacokinetics results, the usual olanzapine dose recommended is 5–10 mg once daily, with a target dose of 10 mg/day as a likely good clinical guideline for most adolescent patients. In cases where the psychosis is resistant to treatment with at least two atypical antipsychotics, it is advised that clozapine be used.

What key messages from new research are not widely being used?

Professor Chris Hollis   The use of atypical antipsychotics for child and adolescent-onset schizophrenia is still inconsistent. These younger patients are likely to derive greatest benefit from these drugs' improved side-effect profile and greater efficacy.

There are still delays in diagnosing schizophrenia in children and adolescents. Recent research suggests that the predictive validity of early diagnosis is high.[134] Diagnostic delay can lead to delays in treatment and providing patient/family education and planning services.

Dr Paramala Santosh   Childhood-onset schizophrenia provides an opportunity to look for more salient risk or etiologic factors in a possibly more homogenous patient population. Early-onset schizophrenia is associated with more severe premorbid neuro-developmental abnormalities, more cytogenetic anomalies (for example, deletion of

131   Frazier J A, Geidd J N, Kaysen D, et al (1996) Childhood-onset schizophrenia: brain magnetic imaging rescan after two years of clozapine maintenance. American Journal of Psychiatry, 153, 564–566.

132   Blumenthal J, Hamburger S, Jeffries N, et al (1999) Progressive cortical change during adolescence in childhood-onset schizophrenia. A longitudinal magnetic resonance imaging study. Archives of General Psychiatry, 56, 649–654.

133   Hollis C P (2000) Adolescent schizophrenia. Advances in Psychiatric Treatment, 6, 83–92.

134   As above.

chromosome 22q11, velocardiofacial syndrome), and potentially greater family histories of schizophrenia and associated spectrum disorders than later-onset cases. Premorbid disturbances in motor/language development have a significant impact on cognitive impairment seen during the course of the illness. Childhood-onset schizophrenia shows progressive ventricular enlargement, reduction in total brain and thalamus volume, changes in temporal lobe structures, and reductions in frontal metabolism.

There are more than 15 studies that have demonstrated antipsychotic efficacy in childhood and adolescent schizophrenia. Atypical antipsychotics should be used as the first-line treatment, along with appropriate psychosocial interventions. Clozapine has a high antipsychotic efficacy during an acute schizophrenic episode, significantly improves negative symptoms, and produces relatively low extrapyramidal symptoms. However, agranulocytosis, weight gain, and hypersalivation are significant side-effects and need regular monitoring.

REFERENCES

● CLINICAL EVIDENCE ●

Lewrie S M & McIntosh A (2000) **Schizophrenia**. In *Clinical Evidence. A Compendium of the Best Available Evidence for Effective Health Care*, Issue 4, pp. 558–577. London: BMJ Publishing Group.

● SYSTEMATIC REVIEWS AND META-ANALYSES ●

Aylward E, Walker E & Bettes B (1984) **Intelligence in schizophrenia: meta-analysis of the research**. *Schizophrenia Bulletin*, **10**, 430–459.

Banaschewski H, Schultz E, Martin M, *et al* (2000) **Cognitive functions and psychopathological symptoms in early-onset schizophrenia**. *European Journal of Child and Adolescent Psychiatry*, **9**, 11–20.

Hollis C & Taylor E (1997) **Schizophrenia: a critique from the developmental psychopathology perspective**. In *Neurodevelopment and Adult Psychopathology* (eds M S Keshervan & R M Murray). Cambridge: Cambridge University Press.

Jacobson L & Rapoport J (1998) **Research update: childhood-onset schizophrenia: implications for clinical and neurobiological research**. *Journal of Child Psychology and Psychiatry*, **39**, 101–113.

Joy C B, Adams C E & Lawrie S M (1998) **Haloperidol for schizophrenia**. Cochrane Review. In *The Cochrane Library*, Issue 1. Oxford: Update Software.

Nicholson R, Lenane M, Hamburger S D, *et al* (2000) **Lessons from childhood-onset schizophrenia**. *Brain Research Review*, **31**, 147–156.

Nicol M M, Robertson L & Connaughton J A (2000) **Life skills programmes for people with chronic mental illness**. Cochrane Review. In *The Cochrane Library*, Issue 4. Oxford: Update Software.

Remschmidt H (1973) **Observations on the role of anxiety in neurotic and psychotic disorders at an early age**. *Journal of Autism and Childhood Schizophrenia*, **3**, 106–114.

——, Fleischaker C, Henninghausen K, *et al* (2000) **Management of schizophrenia in children and adolescents. The role of clozapine**. *Paediatric Drugs*, **2**, 253–262.

Remschmidt H, Hennighausen K & Clement H W (2000) **Atypical neuroleptics in child and adolescent psychiatry**. *European Child and Adolescent Psychiatry*, **9** (suppl.), 19.

Rey J M & Walter G (1997) **Half a century of ECT use in young people**. *American Journal of Psychiatry*, **54**, 595–602.

Sacker A, Done D J & Crow T J (1996) **Obstetric complications in children born to parents with schizophrenia: a meta-analysis of case-control studies**. *Psychological Medicine*, **26**, 279–287.

Srisurapanont M, Disayavanish C & Taimkaew K (1999) **Quetiapine for schizophrenia**. Cochrane Review. In *The Cochrane Library*, Issue 1. Oxford: Update Software.

Tuunainen A & Gilbody S M (2000) **Newer atypical antipsychotic medication versus clozapine for schizophrenia**. Cochrane Review. In *The Cochrane Library*, Issue 4. Oxford: Update Software.

Vita A, Dieci M, Giobbio G M, *et al* (1994) **A reconsideration of the relationship between cerebral structural abnormalities and family history of schizophrenia**. *Psychiatry Research*, **53**, 41–55.

Volkmar F R (1996) **Childhood and adolescent psychosis: a review of the past 10 years**. *Journal of the American Academy of Child and Adolescent Psychiatry*, **35**, 843–851.

● PRACTICE PARAMETERS ●

McCellan J M & Werry J S (1994) **Practice parameters for the assessment and treatment of children and adolescents with schizophrenia**. *Journal of the American Academy of Child and Adolescent Psychiatry*, **33**, 616–635.

● CLINICAL GUIDELINES ●

Frances A, Docherty J P & Kahn D A (eds) (1996) **The expert consensus guideline series: Treatment of schizophrenia**. *Journal of Clinical Psychiatry*, **57** (suppl. 12b).

McEvoy J P, Scheifler P L & Frances A (eds) (1999) **The expert consensus guideline series: Treatment of schizophrenia**. *Journal of Clinical Psychiatry*, **60** (suppl. 11).

● REVIEWS ●

Clark A & Lewis S (1998) **Treatment of schizophrenia in childhood and adolescence**. *Journal of Child Psychology and Psychiatry*, **39**, 1071–1081.

Hollis C P (2000) **Adolescent schizophrenia**. *Advances in Psychiatric Treatment*, **6**, 83–92.

Werry J S & Taylor E (1994) **Schizophrenia and allied disorders**. In ***Child and Adolescent Psychiatry: Modern Approaches*** (eds M Rutter & E Taylor). Oxford: Blackwell Scientific.

● CLASSIC PAPERS ●

Frazier J A, Geidd J N, Kaysen D, *et al* (1996) **Childhood-onset schizophrenia: brain magnetic imaging rescan after two years of clozapine maintenance**. *American Journal of Psychiatry*, **153**, 564–566.

Kallman F J & Roth B (1956) **Genetic aspects of preadolescent schizophrenia**. *American Journal of Psychiatry*, **112**, 599–606.

Kolvin I (1971) **Studies in the childhood psychoses: diagnostic criteria and classification**. *British Journal of Psychiatry*, **118**, 381–384.

Kumra S, Frazier J A, Jacobson L K, *et al* (1996) **Childhood-onset schizophrenia: A double blind clozapine-haloperidol comparison**. *Archives of General Psychiatry*, **38**, 1090–1097.

Rutter M (1972) **Childhood schizophrenia reconsidered**. *Journal of Autism and Childhood Schizophrenia*, **2**, 315–407.

● CUTTING EDGE PAPERS ●

Alaghband-Rad J, Hamburger S D, Giedd J, *et al* (1997) **Childhood-onset schizophrenia: biological markers in relation to clinical characteristics**. *American Journal of Psychiatry*, **154**, 64–68.

Frazier J A, Geidd J N, Kaysen D, *et al* (1996) **Childhood-onset schizophrenia: brain magnetic imaging rescan after two years of clozapine maintenance**. *American Journal of Psychiatry*, **153**, 564–566.

Hollis C (2000) **The adult outcomes of child and adolescent-onset schizophrenia: Diagnostic stability and predictive validity**. *American Journal of Psychiatry*, **157**, 1652–1659.

Kuma S, Frazier J A, Jacobson L K, *et al* (1996) **Childhood-onset schizophrenia: a double blind clozapine-haloperidol comparison**. *Archives of General Psychiatry*, **53**, 1090–1097.

Rapoport J L, Giedd J, Blumenthal J, *et al* (1999) **Progressive cortical change during adolescence in childhood-onset schizophrenia. A longitudinal magnetic resonance imaging study**. *Archives of General Psychiatry*, **56**, 649–664.

● USEFUL WEBSITES ●

Mental Health Foundation http://www.mentalhealth.org.uk

Mind http://www.mind.org.uk

Cochrane Controlled Trials Register
19 hits (keywords: psychosis AND child)
23 hits (keywords: psychosis AND child*)
70 hits (keywords: psychosis AND adolescen*)
102 hits (keywords: schizophrenia AND child*)
463 hits (keywords: schizophrenia AND adolescen*)

Cochrane Depression, Anxiety and Neurosis Group
Contact: Dr Natalie Khin, Review Group Coordinator, New Zealand.
n.khin@suckland.ac.nz

SUBSTANCE MISUSE

INTRODUCTION

Substance misuse refers to the misuse of legal (including prescription medication) and illegal drugs. The substances most commonly abused by adolescents are tobacco, alcohol and cannabis.

At least two-thirds of young people with substance misuse disorders are likely to have co-existing (usually pre-existing) psychosocial problems. Concerns are raised in the literature about the appropriateness of applying adult dependence and misuse criteria to adolescent assessments, and about the shortcomings of current services and treatment programmes for young people with substance misuse problems. Current patterns of polydrug use among young people can complicate assessment, particularly in different youth cultures and among different ethnic groups, and young people who are no longer in formal education are a particular challenge if access to designated services is not available.[135]

The prevalence of drug misuse for the under 18-year-old population is quite difficult to determine. However, prevalence figures from a recent survey of drug use in the UK[136] do include figures for children and adolescents. The survey found that about half of the population of 16–24-year-olds in England and Wales have used illicit drugs and solvents at some point in their lives. This figure dropped slightly in Northern Ireland to approximately 40%. The study also provides a breakdown of prevalence figures according to drug type:

- **Cannabis**: 30–40% of 15–16-year-olds in England, Scotland and Wales reported having used cannabis (this figure rises to nearly half of 16–24-year-olds).

- **Hallucinogens, amphetamines, cocaine and ecstasy**: Approximately 39% of 16–24-year-olds in England and Wales reported ever having taken hallucinogens (defined as LSD, magic mushrooms and amyl nitrite), while the prevalence figures were 21% for amphetamines, 10.7% for ecstasy and 7% for cocaine.

- **Opiates (heroin, methadone)**: Among males, 0.9% of those aged 16–24 years reported using opiates in the past month, compared with 0.5% for females.

DIAGNOSIS AND AETIOLOGY

Substance misuse can be linked to:

- social deprivation and community dysfunction;

- family conflict and dysfunctional parenting; and

- parent and sibling substance misuse.[137]

---

135 Gilvarry E (2000) **Substance abuse in young people**. *Journal of Child Psychology and Psychiatry*, **41**, 55–80.

136 UK Drug Report 2000 –The Drug Situation in the UK. See http://www.drugscope.org.uk/druginfo/report2000.asp

137 Gilvarry E (2000) **Substance abuse in young people**. *Journal of Child Psychology and Psychiatry*, **41**, 55–80.

by Ms Helen Shaw

What developments have there been in the past 2–5 years in the prevention of substance abuse?

The clearer definition of co-existing psychosocial problems has enabled prevention programmes to better reflect the reality of youthful drug use, and has allowed treatment modalities to be more tailored to the complex needs of substance-misusing young people.

Parents, politicians and some health and education professionals may need help to better contextualise drug use and risk, rather than simply scapegoating drug users. Such understandings could lead to more constructive partnerships, better assessment, and the closer integration of service responses.

More rigorous evaluation of the effectiveness of the commonly presented prevention programmes has been a feature of recent developments in the field. Current policies and practice have been slow to reflect this, however, as significant public funds are still spent on universal (one size fits all) programmes with seriously flawed design faults.

REFERENCES

● SYSTEMATIC REVIEWS AND META-ANALYSES ●

Derzon J H & Lipsey M W (1999) **Predicting tobacco use to age 18: A synthesis of longitudinal research**. *Addiction*, **94**, 995–1006.

Elmquist D L (1995) **A systematic review of parent-oriented programs to prevent children's use of alcohol and other drugs**. *Journal of Drug Education*, **25**, 251–279.

Fillmore K M, Hartka E, Johnstone B M, *et al* (1991) **Preliminary results from a meta-analysis of drinking behavior in multiple longitudinal studies**. *British Journal of Addiction*, **86**, 1203–1210.

——, ——, ——, *et al* (1991) **The collaborative alcohol-related longitudinal project: a meta-analysis of life course variation in drinking**. *British Journal of Addiction to Alcohol and Other Drugs*, **86**, 1221–1267.

——, ——, ——, *et al* (1991) **The collaborative alcohol-related longitudinal project: preliminary results from a meta-analysis of drinking behaviour in multiple longitudinal studies**. *British Journal of Addiction to Alcohol and Other Drugs*, **86**, 1203–1210.

Foxcroft D R & Lowe G (1991) **Adolescent drinking behaviour and family socialization factors: a meta-analysis**. *Journal of Adolescence*, **14**, 255–273.

Gowing L, Ali R & White J (2000) **Opioid antagonists and adrenergic agonists for the management of opioid withdrawal**. Cochrane Review. In *The Cochrane Library*, Issue 1. Oxford: Update Software.

——, —— & —— (2000) **Opioid antagonists under sedation or anaesthesia for opioid withdrawal**. Cochrane Review. In *The Cochrane Library*, Issue 4. Oxford: Update software.

Johnstone B M, Leino E V, Ager C R, *et al* (1996) **Determinants of life-course variation in the frequency of alcohol consumption: meta-analysis of studies from the collaborative alcohol-related longitudinal project**. *Journal of Studies on Alcohol*, **57**, 494–506.

Kirchmayer U, Davoli M & Verster A (1999) **Naltrexone maintenance treatment for opioid dependence**. Cochrane Review. In *The Cochrane Library*, Issue 1. Oxford: Update Software. (Refers to all ages.)

Lima A R, Lima M S, Churchill R, *et al* (2001) **Carbamazepine for cocaine dependence**. Cochrane Review. In *The Cochrane Library*, Issue 1. Oxford: Update Software. (Refers to all ages.)

Minozzi S & Grilli R (1997) **The systematic review of studies on the efficacy of interventions for the primary prevention of alcohol abuse among adolescents**. *Epidemiologia e Prevenzione*, **21**, 180–188.

New Zealand Health Technology Assessment (1998) **Adolescent therapeutic day programmes and community-based programmes for serious mental illness and serious drug and alcohol problems: A critical appraisal of the literature**. *NZHTA Report*, **5**, 56.

Osborn D A & Cole M J (2000) **Sedatives for opiate withdrawal in newborn infants**. Cochrane Review. In *The Cochrane Library*, Issue 4. Oxford: Update Software.

Pollock V E (1992) **Meta-analysis of subjective sensitivity to alcohol in sons of alcoholics**. *American Journal of Psychiatry*, **149**, 1534–1538.

Rooney B L & Murray D M (1996) **A meta-analysis of smoking prevention programs after adjustment for errors in the unit of analysis**. *Health Education Quarterly*, **21**, 48–64.

Sowden A J & Arblaster L (2000) **Mass media interventions for preventing smoking in young people**. Cochrane Review. In *The Cochrane Library*, Issue 4. Oxford: Update Software.

—— & —— (2000) **Community interventions for preventing smoking in young people**. Cochrane Review. In *The Cochrane Library*, Issue 4. Oxford: Update Software.

Stanton M D & Shadish W R (1997) **Outcome, attrition, and family-couples treatment for drug abuse: A meta-analysis and review of the controlled, comparative studies**. *Psychological Bulletin*, **122**, 170–191. (Reviewed on DARE.)

Stead M & Hastings G (1995) **Developing options for a programme on adolescent smoking in Wales**. *Health Promotion Wales Technical Report*, **16**, 32.

Sussman S, Lichtman K, Ritt A, *et al* (1999) **Effects of thirty-four adolescent tobacco use cessation and prevention trials on regular users of tobacco products**. *Substance Use and Misuse*, **34**, 1469–1503. (Reviewed on DARE.)

Tobler N (1994) **Meta-analytical issues for prevention intervention research**. *NIDA Research Monographs*, **142**, 342–403.

—— (2000) **Lessons learned**. *Journal of Primary Prevention*, **20**, 261–274.

——, Roona M R, Ochshorn P, *et al* (2000) **School-based adolescent drug prevention programs: 1998 meta-analysis**. *Journal of Primary Prevention*, **20**, 275–336.

White D & Pitts M (1998) **Educating young people about drugs: a systematic review**. *Addiction*, **93**, 1475–1487.

● PRACTICE PARAMETERS ●

American Academy of Child and Adolescent Psychiatry (1997) **Practice parameters for the assessment and treatment of children and adolescents with substance use disorders**. *Journal of the American Academy of Child and Adolescent Psychiatry*, **36** (suppl.), 1405–1565.

American Psychiatric Association (1995) **Practice guideline for treatment of patients with substance use disorders: alcohol, cocaine, opioids**. *American Journal of Psychiatry*, **152** (suppl.), 1–59.

● REVIEWS ●

Allott R, Paxton R & Leonard R (1999) **Drug education: a review of British Government policy and evidence on effectiveness**. *Health Education Research*, **14**, 491–505.

Dusenbury L (2000) **Family-based drug abuse prevention programmes: a review**. *Journal of Primary Prevention*, **20**, 337–352.

Gilvarry E (1998) **Young drug users: early intervention**. *Drugs: Education, Prevention and Policy*, **5**, 281–292.

—— (2000) **Substance abuse in young people**. *Journal of Child Psychology & Psychiatry*, **41**, 55–80.

Lloyd C, Joyce R, Hurry J, *et al* (2000) **The effectiveness of primary school drug education**. *Drugs: Education, Prevention and Policy*, **7**, 109–126.

Meyers K, Hagan T A, Zanis D, *et al* (1999) **Critical issues in adolescent substance use assessment**. *Drug and Alcohol Dependence*, **55**, 235–246.

Najavits L M & Weiss R D (1994) **Variations in therapist effectiveness in the treatment of patients with substance use disorders: an empirical review**. *Addiction*, **89**, 679–688.

Paglia A & Room R (1999) **Preventing substance abuse problems among youth: a literature review and recommendations**. *Journal of Primary Prevention*, **20**, 3–50.

Weinberg N Z, Rahdert E, Colliver J D, *et al* (1998) **Adolescent substance abuse: a review of the past 10 years**. *Journal of the American Academy of Child and Adolescent Psychiatry*, **37**, 252–261.

Zeitlin H (1999) **Psychiatric comorbidity with substance misuse in children and teenagers**. *Drug and Alcohol Dependence*, **55**, 225–234.

● CUTTING EDGE PAPERS ●

Boys A, Marsden J, Fountain J, *et al* (1999) **What influences young people's use of drugs? A qualitative study of decision-making**. *Drugs: Education, Prevention and Policy*, **6**, 373–387.

Geller B (1997) **Double-blind placebo-controlled study of lithium for adolescents with bipolar disorders with secondary substance dependency**. *Journal of the American Academy of Child and Adolescent Psychiatry*, **37**, 171–178.

Stockwell T (1999) **A new agenda for harm minimization?** *Drugs: Education, Prevention and Policy*, **6**, 205–208.

● REPORTS ●

Crome I B, Christian J & Green C (2000) **The development of a unique designated community drug service for adolescents: policy, prevention and education implications**. *Drugs: Education, Prevention and Policy*, **7**, 87–108.

Fergusson D M & Horwood L J (1997) **Early onset cannabis use and psychological adjustment in young adults**. *Addiction*, **92**, 279–296.

Ghelani P (1998) *Volatile Substance Abuse*. Report 160. London: National Children's Bureau.

Hansen W B & McNeal R B (1999) **Drug education practice: results of an observational study**. *Health Education Research*, **14**, 85–97.

Jarvis L (1996) *Smoking Among Secondary School Children in 1996 England*. Office of National Statistics, Social Security Division. London: The Stationery Office.

—— (1996) *Teenage Smoking Attitudes in 1996: A Survey of the Smoking Behaviour, Knowledge and Attitudes of 11 to 15 year olds in England*. Office of National Statistics, Social Security Division. London: The Stationery Office.

Mounteney J (1998) *Children of Drug-using Parents*. Report 163. London: National Children's Bureau.

SCODA and The Children's Legal Centre (1999) *Policy Guidance for Drug Intervention*. London: SCODA.

Wibberley C & Price J F (2000) **Young people's drug use: facts and feelings implications for the normalization debate**. *Drugs: Education, Prevention and Policy*, **7**, 147–162.

Winter K C (1999) *Screening and Assessing Adolescents for Substance Use Disorders*. Treatment Improvement Protocol (TIP) series 31. United States Department of Health and Human Services, Public Health Service, Substance Abuse and Mental Health Services Administration (SAMHSA). Available online at http://hstat.nlm.nih.gov/

Wyvill B & Ives R (2000) **Finding out about young people's ideas on drugs and drug use – methodology**. *Drugs: Education, Prevention and Policy*, **7**, 127–137.

—— & Ives R (2000) **Finding out about young people's ideas on drugs and drug use – applications and limitations**. *Drugs: Education, Prevention and Policy*, **7**, 139–146.

● USEFUL WEBSITES ●

Trashed http://www.trashed.co.uk/index2.html

Web of Addictions http://www.well.com/user/woa

TIC DISORDER: tics and Gilles de la Tourette syndrome

INTRODUCTION

Tics are involuntary, purposeless, repetitive movements. Motor tics are more common in children and often involve the face, neck and arms and other parts of the upper body such as eye-blinking, neck-jerking, shoulder-shrugging and facial grimacing. Tics are usually categorised as simple or complex tics. Tourette's syndrome is characterised by chronic, incapacitating vocal and multiple motor tics and has an onset before the age of 18 years.

Simple tics occur in about 20% of children and are usually transient, although 1% of children may continue to suffer from tics.[138] The ONS survey figures indicate that tic disorders occur in 0.1% of children in Great Britain.[139] Tics have been found to be more common in boys than in girls.[140] Tourette's syndrome, on the other hand, occurs in approximately 0.029% of children according to a survey of English children,[141] but these figures can range from 0.005 to 0.3%.[142]

DIAGNOSIS AND AETIOLOGY

Tics can be distinguished from other forms of motor disorders by:

- the sudden and rapid nature of the movements;
- the movements occurring for no apparent purpose;
- the absence of neurological disorder;
- the repetitive nature; and
- their easy voluntary reproducibility.

The ICD–10 has five categories of tic disorders:

1. transient tics disorder;
2. chronic motor or vocal tic disorder;
3. combined vocal and multiple motor tic disorder (de la Tourette);
4. other tic disorders; and
5. tic disorder, unspecified.

The DSM–IV–TR categories of tics are very similar, however category 3 above is called Tourette's disorder and categories 4 and 5 above fall under Tic disorder not otherwise specified.

---

138 Shapiro & Shapiro (1981) cited in Berelowitz M & Nelki J (1993) Clinical syndrome in middle childhood. In *Seminars in Child and Adolescent Psychiatry* (eds D Black & D Cottrell), pp. 124–153. London: Gaskell.

139 Meltzer H, Gatward R, Goodman R, *et al* (2000) *The Mental Health of Children and Adolescents in Great Britain*. London: The Stationery Office.

140 Wallace W A, Crown J M, Berger M, *et al* (1997) *Child and Adolescent Mental Health: Health Care Needs Assessment. The Epidemiologically Based Needs Assessment Reviews* (eds A Stevens & J Raftery). 2nd series. Oxon: Radcliffe Medical Press Ltd.

141 Kurtz Z, Thornes R & Wolkind S (1996) *Services for the Mental Health of Children and Young People in England: Assessment of Needs and Unmet Needs*. London: South West Thames Regional Health Authority.

142 American Psychiatric Association (2000) *Diagnostic and Statistical Manual of Mental Disorders*. 4th edn (DSM–IV–TR). Washington DC: APA.

Although motor and vocal tics are necessary for the diagnosis of Tourette's syndrome other characteristic features include echolia, echopraxia and palilalia, which occur in a substantial number of patients; coprolalia is less common, occurring in less than one-third of clinical cohorts and fewer children and family members.[143] Tourette's syndrome is also associated with disorders such as ADHD, OCD, self-injurious behaviours, depression, anxiety and personality disorder.[144] In a recent study embracing 3,500 clinic patients with Tourette's syndrome from 22 countries,[145] the vast majority (around 85%) had comorbid psychopathology and associated behaviours. It is of little surprise that in the first investigation systematically studying the quality of life (QOL) of patients with Tourette's syndrome, that QOL was significantly worse than in a general population sample.[146] Factors influencing the QOL domains in the study were employment status, tic severity, obsessive–compulsive behaviour, anxiety and depression.

It has been suggested that tics may have a neurological, chemical and genetic basis and seem to be aggravated by emotional stress.

Tourette's syndrome has a genetic basis, although other factors in aetiology have been suggested, such as pregnancy or birth difficulties, as well as streptoccoal infections. Tourette's syndrome was once thought to be very uncommon, but recent studies have suggested a prevalence of no less than between 1%[147] of children in Sweden and 2.9%[148] of school children in the UK. The prevalence of Tourette's syndrome in people with learning difficulties of a variety of kinds[149] including autistic spectrum disorders[150] is even higher.

CRITICAL QUESTIONS

by Professor Mary Robertson

What developments have there been in the management of Tourette's syndrome in the past 2–5 years?

The treatment of Tourette's syndrome is, in a word, complex. If the individual is mildly affected, reassurance and psychoeducation of the patient and family may well be all that is required. If the patient has predominantly motor and vocal tics,

143 Robertson M M (1994) **Annotation: Gilles de la Tourette syndrome – an update.** *Journal of Child Psychology and Psychiatry*, **35**, 597–611.
144 Robertson M M (2000) **Invited review. Tourette syndrome, associated conditions and the complexities of treatment.** *Brain*, **123**, 425–462.
   Robertson M M *et al* (1997) **Personality disorder and psychopathology in Tourette's syndrome: A controlled study.** *British Journal of Psychiatry*, **171**, 283–286.
145 Freeman R D (2000) **An international perspective on Tourette syndrome; selected findings from 3,500 individuals in 22 countries.** *Developmental Medicine and Child Neurology*, **42**, 436–447.
146 Elstner K, Selai C E, Trimbale M R, *et al* (2001) **Quality of Life (QOL) of patients with Gilles de la Tourette's syndrome.** *Acta Psychiatrica Scandinavica*, **103**, 52–59.
147 Kadesjo B & Gillberg C (2000) **Tourette's disorder: Epidemiology and comorbidity in primary school children.** *Journal of the American Academy of Child and Adolescent Psychiatry*, **39**, 548–555.
148 Mason A *et al* (1989) **The prevalence of Tourette syndrome in a mainstream school population.** *Developmental Medicine and Child Neurology*, **40**, 292–296.
149 Eapen V, Robertson M M, Zeitlin H, *et al* (1997) **Gilles de la Tourette's syndrome in special education.** *Journal of Neurology*, **244**, 378–382.
150 Baron-Cohen S, Mortimore C, Moriarty J, *et al* (1999) **The prevalence of Gilles de la Tourette syndrome in children and adolescents with autism.** *Journal of Child Psychology and Psychiatry*, **40**, 213–218.

antipsychotics/neuroleptics are still the mainstay of treatment, with haloperidol and pimozide widely used in the USA, and sulpiride and tiapride in Europe. Some of the 'atypicals', including risperidone and olanzapine have been documented as useful. If ADHD is prominent, clonidine or methylphenidate may be useful, but the latter may increase tics. If OCD is prominent, an SSRI plus a neuroleptic is suggested. The aggression and rage are often difficult to treat, and may require combination strategies.

Immunomodulatory, antibiotic, antiviral and hormonal therapy have all been noted to be useful in a small number of patients, but these treatments remain speculative, and are not recommended for the general psychiatrist. Psychosurgery has also been used, but is not suggested outside a specialist centre.

Psychotherapy is important and helps with general well-being, but does not help the tics as such. Often, specialists write to schools giving guidelines that might help in the educational setting.

What are the key messages from new research that are not being widely used?

It is now generally recognised that Tourette's syndrome is genetic, although streptococcal infections may be aetiological in a subgroup of patients. Perinatal infections are also implicated in the aetiopathogenesis. A few specialist centres are examining these aspects, but to date there are no treatment implications as such. The search for an endophenotype continues and, when found, may well have treatment implications in the future.

Neuroimaging abnormalities have been demonstrated that confirm the primary biological nature of the disorder. Stress, however, can also make symptoms worse. It is therefore important to have a holistic approach to treatment. Thus, psychoeducation and supportive psychotherapy are very important and it is useful, where possible, to involve family members in these aspects of treatment.

REFERENCES

● SYSTEMATIC REVIEWS AND META-ANALYSES ●

None identified.

● CLINICAL GUIDELINES ●

None identified.

● REVIEWS ●

Kurlan R (1999) **Investigating Tourette syndrome as a neurological sequela of rheumatic fever**. *CNS Spectrums*, **4**, 62–67.

Leckman J F, Peterson B S, Anderson G M, *et al* (1997) **Pathogenesis of Tourette's syndrome**. *Journal of Child Psychology and Psychiatry*, **38**, 119–142.

Patel P I (1996) **Quest for the elusive genetic basis of Tourette syndrome (editorial)**. *American Journal of Human Genetics*, **59**, 980–982.

—— (1994) **Annotation: Gilles de la Tourette syndrome – an update**. *Journal of Child Psychology and Psychiatry*, **35**, 597–611.

—— (2000) **Invited review. Tourette syndrome, associated conditions and the complexities of treatment**. *Brain*, **123**, 425–462.

● CLASSIC PAPERS ●

Bliss J (1980) **Sensory experiences of Gilles de la Tourette syndrome**. *Archives of General Psychiatry*, **37**, 1343–1347.

Bruun R D, Shapiro A K, Shapiro E, *et al* (1976) **A follow-up of 78 patients with Gilles de la Tourette syndrome**. *American Journal of Psychiatry*, **30**, 392–396.

Gilles de la Tourette G (1885) **Etude sur une affection nerveuse caracterisee par de l'incoordination motrice accompagnee d'echolalie et de coprolalie**. *Archive in Neurology*, **9**, 19–42, 158–200.

Sacks O (1995) **A surgeon's life**. In *An Anthropologist on Mars*. New York: Knopf; London: Picador.

● CUTTING EDGE PAPERS ●

Baron-Cohen S, Mortimore C, Moriarty J, *et al* (1999) **The prevalence of Gilles de la Tourette syndrome in children and adolescents with autism: A large scale study**. *Psychological Medicine*, **29**, 1151–1159.

Eapen V, Robertson M M, Alsobrook II J P, *et al* (1997) **Obsessive compulsive disorder in Gilles de la Tourette syndrome and obsessive compulsive disorder: differences by diagnosis and family history**. *American Journal of Medical Genetics (Neuropsychiatric Genetics)*, **74**, 432–438.

Pauls D L, Leckman J F & Cohen D J (1994) **Evidence against a genetic relationship between Tourette's syndrome and anxiety, depression, panic and phobic disorders**. *British Journal of Psychiatry*, **164**, 215–221.

Swedo S E, Leonard H L, Garvey M, *et al* (1998) **Pediatric auto-immune neuropsychiatric disorders associated with streptococcal infections: clinical description of the first 50 cases**. *American Journal of Psychiatry*, **155**, 264–271.

The Tourette Syndrome Association International Consortium for Genetics (1999) **A complete genome scan in sib-pairs affected with Gilles de la Tourette syndrome**. *American Journal of Human Genetics*, **65**, 1428–1436.

● BOOKS ●

Carroll A & Robertson M (2000) *Tourette Syndrome: A Practical Guide for Teachers, Parents and Carers*. London: David Fulton Publishers.

Kushner H I (1999) *A Cursing Brain? The Histories of Tourette Syndrome*. Massachusetts: Harvard University Press.

Leckman J F & Cohen D J (1999) *Tourette's Syndrome – Tics, Obsessions, Compulsions. Developmental Psychopathology and Clinical care*. Chichester: John Wiley & Sons.

Robertson M M & Eapen V (1995) *Movement and Allied disorders in Childhood*. Chichester: John Wiley & Sons.

—— & Baron-Cohen S (1998) *Tourette Syndrome: The Facts*. Oxford: Oxford University Press.

● FURTHER READING ●

Apter A, Pauls D L, Bleich A, *et al* (1993) **An epidemiological study of Gilles de la Tourette syndrome in Israel**. *Archives of General Psychiatry*, **9**, 734–738.

Cohen D J (1991) **Tourette's syndrome: a model disorder for integrating psychoanalysis and biological perspectives**. *International Review of Psychoanalysis*, **18**, 195–209.

Elstner K, Selai C E, Trimble M R, *et al* (2001) **Quality of life (QOL) of patients with Gilles de la Tourette's syndrome**. *Acta Psychiatrica Scandinavica*, **103**, 52–59.

Leckman J F, Dolnasky E S & Hardin M T (1990) **Perinatal factors in the expression of Tourette's syndrome: an exploratory study**. *Journal of the American Academy of Child and Adolescent Psychiatry*, **29**, 220–206.

Pauls D L, Pakstis A J & Kurlan R (1990) **Segregation and linkage analysis of Gilles de la Tourette syndrome and related disorders**. *Journal of the American Academy of Child and Adolescent Psychiatry*, **29**, 195–203.

Robertson M M & Reinstein D Z (1991) **Convulsive tic disorder. Georges Gilles de la Tourette, Guinon and Grasset on the phenomenology and psychopathology of the Gilles de la Tourette Syndrome**. *Behavioural Neurology*, **4**, 29–56.

——, Banerjee S, Fox-Hiley P J, *et al* (1997) **Personality disorder and psychopathology in Tourette's syndrome: A controlled study**. *British Journal of Psychiatry*, **171**, 283–286.

Simkin B (1992) **Mozart's scatalogical disorder**. *British Medical Journal*, **305**, 1563–1567.

Stern J S & Robertson M M (1997) **Tics associated with autistic and pervasive developmental disorders (review)**. *Neurological Clinics*, **15**, 345–355.

Wilensky A (2000) ***Passing for Normal***. London: Simon & Schuster.

Cochrane Controlled Trials Register
0 hits (keywords: tourette's syndrome*)
86 hits (keywords: tourett* syndrome*)
38 hits (keywords: tics AND child*)

Cochrane Movement Disorders Group
Contact: Dr Joaquim Ferreire, Review Group Coordinator, Lisbon, Portugal.
Tel: +351 1797 3453. Movementdisord@mail.telepac.pt

Section 6: treatment approaches

PSYCHOTHERAPEUTIC APPROACHES

INTRODUCTION

There are many forms of psychotherapy such as cognitive–behavioural therapy (CBT), family therapy, group therapy, psychodynamic therapy and music therapy. The type of approach to therapy may depend on the developmental stage of the child. For example, various forms of play therapy are commonly used in younger children, with older children being involved in talking therapies. Essential to all individual psychotherapy is the therapy environment, in which a relationship of trust between the therapist and young person needs to develop for the therapy to be effective.[151]

● COGNITIVE–BEHAVIOURAL THERAPY ●

Cognitive–behavioural therapy combines the use of techniques from cognitive therapy and behavioural therapy. CBT is based on the premise that cognition is a primary determinant of behaviour and mood. Thus, CBT uses behavioural and verbal techniques to identify and correct problematic thinking patterns that are at the root of dysfunctional behaviour.[152]

● FAMILY THERAPY ●

Family therapy is based on the principles of a systemic approach. Difficulties are viewed as developing within a context or pattern of relationships.[153] The focus of intervention is the significant relational network which may be the family or wider social networks. The goal in family therapy reflects a fit between presenting difficulties, context of referral, goals agreed with the family member(s) and organisational context.

An important clinical contribution of family therapy is the development of techniques for convening family meetings and facilitating therapeutic conversations that take into account the diversity of family forms and accompanying beliefs in our multi-cultural society.

● GROUP THERAPY ●

Group therapy is based on the notion that difficulties develop within a network of relationships and not with the individual in isolation. Group therapy explores the relationships within a dynamically changing group, allows for mutual sharing and

---

151 Trowell J (1985) **Individual and group psychotherapy**. In *Child and Adolescent Psychiatry: Modern Approaches* (eds M Rutter, E Taylor & L Hersov). 3rd edn. Oxford: Blackwell Scientific Publications.

152 Medline database.

153 Gorrell Barnes J (1985) **Family therapy**. In *Child and Adolescent Psychiatry: Modern Approaches* (eds M Rutter, E Taylor & L Hersov). 3rd edn. Oxford: Blackwell Scientific Publications.

126

gives a different perspective of common difficulties by being with people with similar problems, as well as an opportunity to obtain feedback from peers.[154]

Groups provide a peer group experience, where the members can experiment being someone different from the person they perceive themselves to be in other group situations such as the family, the neighbourhood 'gang', school or college. Members can explore attitudes towards authority, dependency and nurturing, while giving and receiving feedback that may challenge their self-perceptions and improve relational ties. The group is a microcosm of society, but one that is highly supported, more manageable and potentially less anxiety-provoking. It provides a context for learning social, academic, play and interpersonal skills.

Groups require clear objectives, limits and boundaries to which the members and therapists subscribe. Groups can use a range of different frameworks and mediums, from the agenda-less therapy group to the highly structured and focused 'talking group', as well as groups that include the use of materials like wood, paint, clay, music and dance. Groups may be open, admitting new members as necessary, or closed and time-limited.

● PSYCHODYNAMIC THERAPY ●

Psychodynamic therapy is a method of psychological treatment derived from psychoanalytic theory. This form of therapy focuses on the interplay between mental and emotional forces and how these may affect behaviour.[155]

● MUSIC THERAPY ●

Music therapy uses music as a non-verbal channel of communication to express emotions and verbalise feelings, and to encourage group interactions.[156] The universality of response to musical expression and the musical parameters of emotional communication (as revealed in infancy research)[157] suggest that musicality is innate and, with its temporal and other aesthetic phenomena, has an important role in regulating emotional states in social interaction.[158] Case studies with a wide range of clinical populations attest to the robustness of human capacity for communicative musicality despite handicap, injury or illness.

Music therapy involves the creative use of music to form a therapeutic relationship, in which the child's or adolescent's feelings may be engaged and supported by music in such a way as to develop a sounder sense of self, increase awareness,

---

154 Trowell J (1985) Individual and group psychotherapy. In *Child and Adolescent Psychiatry: Modern Approaches* (eds M Rutter, E Taylor & L Hersov). 3rd edn. Oxford: Blackwell Scientific Publications.

155 Marzillier J & Hall J (1999) *What is Clinical Psychology?* 3rd edn. Oxford: Oxford University Press.

156 Trowell J (1985) Individual and group psychotherapy. In *Child and Adolescent Psychiatry: Modern Approaches* (eds M Rutter, E Taylor & L Hersov). 3rd edn. Oxford: Blackwell Scientific Publications.

157 Papousek H & Papousek M (1981) Musical elements in infants' vocalization: their significance for communication, cognition and creativity. *Advances in Infancy Research*, 1, 163–224.
Trevarthen C (1999) Musicality and the intrinsic motive pulse: Evidence from human psychobiology and infant communication. *Musicae Scientiae,* August, 157–213.

158 Trehub S (2000) Human Processing Predispositions and Musical Universals; Dissanayake E (2000) Antecedents of the Temporal Arts in Early Mother-Infant Interaction
Imberty M (2000) The Question of Innate Competencies in Musical Communication in The Origins of Music (eds N L Wallin, B Merker & S Brown). Cambridge: MIT Press.

motivate, and improve well-being. Normal therapeutic boundaries, including regularity of time and place, are observed.

Developmental and psychodynamic concerns are part of the music therapy process. Music is used improvisationally to meet the child's mood(s), tonal and rhythmic responses, thereby reaching underlying feelings and developing communication and play. Music therapy is used to address many areas of emotional experience, which may include developmental and psychological components, such as sensory and spatial awareness, motor coordination, concentration, preverbal and non-verbal forms of communication, or more complex aspects of emotions and relationship in psychopathological conditions.

GENERAL PSYCHOTHERAPY

● SYSTEMATIC REVIEWS AND META-ANALYSES ●

Bacaltchuk J, Hay P & Trefiglio R (2001) **Antidepressants and psychotherapies for bulimia nervosa**. Protocol for Cochrane Review. In *The Cochrane Library*, Issue 1. Oxford: Update Software.

Harrington R, Whittaker J & Shoebridge P (1998) **Psychological treatment of depression in children and adolescents: A review of treatment research**. *British Journal of Psychiatry*, **173**, 291–298. (Reviewed on DARE.)

Hartmann A, Herzog T & Drinkman A (1992) **Psychotherapy of bulimia nervosa: what is effective? a meta-analysis**. *Journal of Psychosomatic Research*, **2**, 159–167.

Hay P J & Bacaltchuk J (2000) **Psychotherapy for bulimia nervosa and binging**. Cochrane Review. In *The Cochrane Library*, Issue 4. Oxford: Update Software.

Heekerens H P (1989) **Effectiveness of child and adolescent psychotherapy within the scope of meta-analysis**. *Zeitschrift für Kinder und Jugend-psychiatrie*, **17**, 150–157. (Reviewed on DARE.)

Kibby M Y, Tyc V L & Mulhern R K (1998) **Effectiveness of psychological intervention for children and adolescents with chronic medical illness: a meta-analysis**. *Clinical Psychology Review*, **18**, 103–117. (Reviewed on DARE.)

Lewinsohn P M & Clarke G N (1999) **Psychosocial treatments for adolescent depression**. *Clinical Psychology Review*, **19**, 329–342.

Petermann F & Bochmann F (1993) **Metaanalyse von inderverhaltens-trainings: Eine erste Bilanz/Meta-analysis in child behavior therapy: First results**. *Zeitschrift-feur-Klinische-Psychologie*, **22**, 137–152.

Ritter M & Low K G (1996) **Effects of dance/movement therapy: A meta-analysis**. *Arts in Psychotherapy*, **23**, 249–260.

Ritvo R & Papilsky S B (1999) **Effectiveness of psychotherapy**. *Current Opinion in Pediatrics*, **11**, 323–327.

——, Al Mateen C, Ascherman L, *et al* (1999) **Report of the Psychotherapy Task Force of the American Academy of Child and Adolescent Psychiatry**. *Journal of Psychotherapy Practice and Research*, **8**, 93–102.

Russell R L, Greenwald S & Shirk S R (1991) **Language change in child psychotherapy: a meta-analytic review**. *Journal of Consulting and Clinical Psychology*, **59**, 916–919. (Reviewed on DARE.)

Shirk S R & Russell R L (1992) **A reevaluation of estimates of child therapy effectiveness**. *Journal of the American Academy of Child and Adolescent Psychiatry*, **31**, 703–709.

Tillitski C J (1990) **A meta-analysis of estimated effect sizes for group versus individual versus control treatments**. *International Journal of Group Psychotherapy*, **40**, 215–224.

Weiss B & Weisz J R (1990) **The impact of methodological factors on child psychotherapy outcome research: a meta-analysis for researchers**. *Journal of Consulting and Clinical Psychology*, **54**, 789–795.

— & — (1995) **Relative effectiveness of behavioral versus nonbehavioral child psychotherapy**. *Journal of Consulting and Clinical Psychology*, **63**, 317–320.

Weisz J R, Weiss B, Alicke M D, *et al* (1987) **Effectiveness of psychotherapy with children and adolescents: A meta-analysis for clinicians**. *Journal of Consulting and Clinical Psychology*, **55**, 542–549. (Reviewed on DARE.)

—, — & Donenberg G R (1992) **The lab versus the clinic. Effects of child and adolescent psychotherapy**. *American Psychologist*, **47**, 1578–1585.

—, —, Morton T, *et al* (1992) *Meta-analysis of Psychotherapy Outcome Research with Children and Adolescents*. Unpublished manuscript, Los Angeles: University of California.

—, Donenberg G R, Han S S, *et al* (1995) **Bridging the gap between laboratory and clinic in child and adolescent psychotherapy**. *Journal of Consulting and Clinical Psychology*, **63**, 688–701.

—, Weiss B, Han S S, *et al* (1995) **Effects of psychotherapy with children and adolescents revisited: a meta-analysis of treatment outcome studies**. *Psychological Bulletin,* **117**, 450–468.

● REVIEWS ●

Barnett R J, Docherty J P & Frommelt G M (1991) **A review of psychotherapy research since 1963**. *Journal of the American Academy of Child and Adolescent Psychiatry*, **30**, 1–14.

Mitchell J E (1991) **A review of the controlled trials of psychotherapy for bulimia nervosa**. *Journal of Psychosomatic Research*, **35**, 23–31.

Najavits L M & Weiss R D (1994) **Variations in therapist effectiveness in the treatment of patients with substance use disorders: an empirical review**. *Addiction*, **89**, 679–688.

Pearsall D F (1997) **Psychotherapy outcome research in child psychiatric disorders**. *Canadian Journal of Psychiatry*, **42**, 595–601.

Weiss B, Catron T, Harris V, *et al* (1994) **The effectiveness of traditional child psychotherapy**. *Journal of Consulting and Clinical Psychology*, **67**, 82–94.

● REPORTS ●

Russell R L, Greenwald S & Shirk S R (1991) **Language change in child psychotherapy: a meta-analytic review.** *Journal of Consulting and Clinical Psychology*, **59**, 916–919.

● SYSTEMATIC REVIEWS AND META-ANALYSES ●

Baer R A & Nietzel M T (1991) **Cognitive and behavioral treatment of impulsivity in children: A meta-analytic review of the outcome literature**. *Journal of Clinical Child Psychology*, **20**, 400–412.

Bennett D S & Gibbons T A (2000) **Efficacy of child cognitive–behavioral interventions for antisocial behavior: A meta-analysis**. *Child and Family Behavior Therapy*, **22**, 1–15.

Durlak J A, Fuhrman T & Lampman C (1991) **Effectiveness of cognitive behavioural therapy for maladaptive children: a meta-analysis**. *Psychological Bulletin*, **110**, 204–214.

Dush D M, Hirt M L & Schroeder H E (1989) **Self-statement modification in the treatment of child behaviour disorders: a meta-analysis**. *Psychological Bulletin*, **106**, 97–106.

Harrington R, Campbell F, Shoebridge P, *et al* (1998) **Meta-analysis of CBT for depression in adolescents [letter; comment]**. *Journal of the American Academy of Child and Adolescent Psychiatry*, **37**, 1005–1007.

——, Whittaker J, Shoebridge P, *et al* (1998) **Systematic review of efficacy of cognitive behaviour therapies in childhood and adolescent depressive disorder**. *British Medical Journal*, **316**, 1559–1563.

Macdonald G, Ramchandani P, Higgins J, *et al* (2000) **Cognitive–behavioural interventions for sexually abused children**. Protocol for Cochrane Review. In *The Cochrane Library*, Issue 4. Oxford: Update Software.

March J S (1995) **Cognitive–behavioural psychotherapy for children and adolescents with OCD: a review and recommendations for treatment.** *Journal of the American Academy of Child and Adolescent Psychiatry*, **34**, 7–18.

Reinecke M A, Ryan N & DuBois D L (1998) **Cognitive–behavioural therapy of depression and depressive symptoms during adolescence: a review and meta-analysis**. *Journal of the American Academy of Child and Adolescent Psychiatry*, **37**, 26–34.

——, —— & —— (1998) **'Meta-analysis of CBT for depression in adolescents': Dr Reinecke et al reply**. *Journal of the American Academy of Child and Adolescent Psychiatry*, **37**, 1006–1007.

● REVIEWS ●

Harrington R, Whittaker J & Shoebridge P (1998) **Psychological treatment of depression in children and adolescents: a review of treatment research**. *British Journal of Psychiatry*, **173**, 291–298.

Indoe D (1995) **Cognitive behavioural therapy and children of the code**. *Educational and Child Psychology*, **12**, 71–81.

Target M & Fonagy P (1996) **The psychological treatment of child and adolescent psychiatric disorders**. In *What Works for Whom?* (eds A Roth & P Fonagy). London: Guildford Press.

● CUTTING EDGE PAPERS ●

Brent D, Holder D, Kolko D, *et al* (1997) **A clinical psychotherapy trial for adolescent depression comparing cognitive, family and supportive treatments**. *Archives of General Psychiatry*, **54**, 877–885.

Kendell P C (1994) **Treating anxiety disorders in children: results of a randomized clinical trial**. *Journal of Consulting and Clinical Psychology*, **62**, 100–110.

Treasure J L, Katzman M, Schmidt U, *et al* (1999) **Engagement and outcome in the treatment of bulimia nervosa: first phase of a sequential design comparing motivational enhancement therapy and cognitive behavioural therapy**. *Behaviour Research and Therapy*, **37**, 405–418.

Wood A J, Harrington R C & Moore A (1996) **Controlled trial of a brief cognitive–behavioural intervention in adolescent patients with depression**. *Journal of Child Psychology and Psychiatry*, **37**, 727–746.

● REPORTS ●

Best L & Stevens A (1996) *Cognitive Behavioural Therapy in the Treatment of Chronic Fatigue Syndrome*. Development and Evaluation Committee (Report 50). Southampton: Wessex Institute for Health Research and Development.

Royal College of Psychiatrists (1997) *Guidelines to Good Practice in the Use of Behavioural and Cognitive Treatments: Report of a Working Party of the Royal College of Psychiatrists*. London: Royal College of Psychiatrists.

● BOOKS ●

Braswell L & Bloomquist M (1991) *Cognitive Behavioural Therapy with ADHD Children: Child, Family and School Interventions*. New York: Guilford Press.

Graham P (ed.) (1998) *Cognitive–Behavioural Therapy for Children and Families*. Cambridge: Cambridge University Press.

Kendall P C (ed.) (1991) *Child and Adolescent Therapy: Cognitive Behavioural Procedures*. New York: Guilford Press.

Meyers A M & Craighead W E (eds) (1984) *Cognitive Behaviour Therapy with Children*. New York: Plenum Press.

FAMILY THERAPY

● SYSTEMATIC REVIEWS AND META-ANALYSES ●

Carr A (2000) **Evidence-based practice in family therapy and systemic consultation: I: Child-focused problems**. *Journal of Family Therapy*, **22**, 29–60.

Glenny A M, O'Meara S, Melville A, *et al* (1997) **The treatment and prevention of obesity: a systematic review of the literature**. *International Journal of Obesity and Related Metabolic Disorder*s, **21**, 715–737.

Heekerens H P (1991) **Evaluation of family therapy. What is the value of a new treatment approach in paediatric and adolescent problems?** *Acta Paedopsychiatrica*, **54**, 56–67.

Heneghan A M, Horwitz S M & Leventhal J M (1996) **Evaluating intensive family preservation programs: a methodological review**. *Pediatrics*, **97**, 535–542.

Mari J J & Streiner D (1996) **Family intervention reduces relapse rates, rehospitalisation, and costs and increases compliance with medication in schizophrenia**. Cochrane Review. In *The Cochrane Library*, Issue 1. Oxford: Update Software.

Markus E, Lange A & Petigrew T F (1990) **Effectiveness of family therapy: a meta-analysis**. *Journal of Family Therapy*, **12**, 205–221.

Panton J & White E A (1999) **Family therapy for asthma in children**. Cochrane Review. In *The Cochrane Library*, Issue 4. Oxford: Update Software.

Shadish W R, Ragsdaly K, Glaser, R R, *et al* (1995) **The efficacy and effectiveness of marital and family therapy: a perspective from meta-analysis**. *Journal of Marital and Family Therapy,* **21**, 345–360.

Stanton M D & Shadish W R (1997) **Outcome, attrition, and family-couples treatment for drug abuse: A meta-analysis and review of the controlled, comparative studies**. *Psychological Bulletin*, **122**, 170–191.

Woolfenden S, Williams K & Peat J (2001) **Family and parenting interventions in children and adolescents with conduct disorder and delinquency aged 10–17**. Cochrane Review. In *The Cochrane Library*, Issue 2. Oxford: Update Software.

● REVIEWS ●

Chamberlain P & Rosicky J G (1995) **The effectiveness of family therapy in the treatment of adolescents with conduct disorders and delinquency**. *Journal of Marital and Family Therapy,* **21**, 441–459.

Estrada A U & Pinsof W M (1995) **The effectiveness of family therapies for selected behavioural disorders of childhood**. *Journal of Marital and Family Therapy*, **21**, 403–440.

Heekerens H P (1991) **Evaluation of family therapy. What is the value of a new treatment approach in paediatric and adolescent problems?** *Acta Paedopsychiatrica*, **54**, 56–67.

Pinsof W & Wynne L (1995) **The efficacy of marital and family therapy: an empirical overview, conclusions and recommendations**. *Journal of Marital and Family Therapy*, **21**, 585–613.

Waldron H B (1997) **Adolescent substance abuse and family therapy outcome. A review of randomised trials**. *Advances in Clinical Psychology*, **19**, 199–234.

● CLASSIC PAPERS ●

Andersen T (1987) **The reflecting-team: dialogue and meta-dialogue in clinical work.** *Family Process*, **26**, 415–428.

Selvini Palazolli M, Boscolo L, Cecchin G, *et al* (1980) **Hypothesizing–Circularity–Neurality: three guidelines for the conductor of the session**. *Family Process*, **19**, 3–12.

● CUTTING EDGE PAPERS ●

Essex S & Gumbleton J (1999) **'Similar but different' conversations: Working with denial in cases of severe child abuse.** *Australian and New Zealand Journal of Family Therapy*, **20**, 61.

Gorell Barnes G (1999) **Divorce transitions: Identifying risk and promoting resilience for children and their parental relationships**. *Journal of Marital and Family Therapy*, **25**, 425–441.

● PRACTICE CONSIDERATIONS ●

Goldberg D & Hodges M (1992) **The poison of racism and the self-poisoning of adolescents**. *Journal of Family Therapy,* **14**, 51–68.

Huffington C (1999) **Containing failure: consultancy to a residential centre for adolescents**. *Clinical Child Psychiatry and Psychology*, **4**, 533–541.

Reder P (1986) **Multi-agency family systems**. *Journal of Family Therapy,* **8**, 139–152.

Tuffnell G (1993) **Judgements of Solomon: the relevance of a systems approach to psychiatric court reports in child care cases**. *Journal of Family Therapy*, **15**, 413–432.

Usher J M (1991) **Family and couples therapy with gay and lesbian clients: acknowledging the forgotten minority**. *Journal of Family Therapy*, **13**, 131–148.

White M (1984) **Pseudo-encopresis: from avalanche to victory, from vicious to virtuous cycles**. *Family Systems Medicine*, **2**, 150–160.

● BOOKS ●

Dallos R & Draper R (2000) *An Introduction to Family Therapy: Systemic Theory and Practice*. Buckingham: Open University Press.

Gorell Barnes G (1998) *Family Therapy in Changing Times*. London: Macmillan Press.

Wilson J (1998) *Child-Focused Practice: A Collaborative Systemic Approach*. London: Karnac Books.

GROUP THERAPY

● SYSTEMATIC REVIEWS AND META-ANALYSES ●

Dalal F (1997) **A transcultural perspective on psychodynamic psychotherapy addressing internal and external realities**. *Group Analysis*, **30**, 203–215.

de Jong T L & Gorey K M (1996) **Short-term versus long-term group work with female survivors of childhood sexual abuse: A brief meta-analytic review**. *Social Work with Groups*, **19**, 19–27.

Everly G S, Boyle S H & Lating J M (1999) **The effectiveness of psychological debriefing with vicarious trauma: A meta-analysis**. *Stress Medicine*, **15**, 229–233.

Hoag M J & Burlingame G M (1997) **Evaluating effectiveness of child and adolescent group treatment: a meta-analytic review**. *Journal of Clinical Child Psychology*, **26**, 234–246. (Reviewed on DARE.)

Hyde K (1988) **Analytic group psychotherapies**. In *Group Therapy in Britain* (eds M Areline & W Dryden), pp. 13–42. Milton Keynes: Open University Press.

Reeker J, Ensing D & Elliott R (1997) **A meta-analytic investigation of group treatment outcomes for sexually abused children**. *Child Abuse and Neglect*, **21**, 669–680.

● PRACTICE PARAMETERS ●

Brown R, Domingo-Perez L & Murphy D (1989) **Treating impossible children: a therapeutic group on a children's ward**. *Group Analysis*, **22**, 283–298.

del Balzo V & Judges T (1998) **Toward socialisation: the seriously disturbed adolescent in group psychotherapy**. *Group Analysis*, **31**, 157–171.

Woods J (ed.) (1996) **Group analysis with children, families and young people**. *Group Analysis*, **29**, 5–98.

● REVIEWS ●

Dishion T J, McCord J & Toulin F (1999) **When interventions harm: peer group and problem behaviour**. *American Psychologist*, **54**, 755–764.

● CLASSIC PAPERS ●

Cox M (1973) **Group psychotherapy as a redefining process**. *International Journal of Group Psychotherapy*, **23**, 465–473.

Harrison T & Clarke D (1992) **The Northfield experiments**. *British Journal of Psychiatry*, **160**, 698–708.

Pines M (ed.) (1983) **The contribution of S. H. Foulkes to group therapy**. In *The Evolution of Group Analysis*, pp. 265–285. London: Routledge and Kegan Paul.

● CUTTING EDGE PAPERS ●

Davidson B (1999) **Writing as a tool of reflective practice. Sketches and reflections from inside the split milieu of an eating disorders unit**. *Group Analysis*, **32**, 109–124.

Nitsun M (1991) **The anti-group: destructive forces in the group and their therapeutic potential**. *Group Analysis*, **24**, 7–20.

Wood D (1999) **From silent scream to shared sadness**. *Group Analysis*, **32**, 53–70.

● BOOKS ●

Barnes B, Ernst S & Hyde K (1999) ***An Introduction to Groupwork***. London: Macmillan Press.

Dwivedi K N (1993) *Groupwork with Children and Adolescents*. London: Jessica Kingsley.

Kennard D, Roberts J & Winter D A (1993) *A Work Book of Group Analytic Interventions*. London: Routledge.

PSYCHODYNAMIC THERAPY

● SYSTEMATIC REVIEWS ●

Barrows P (1997) **Parent–infant psychotherapy: a review article**. *Journal of Child Psychotherapy*, **23**, 255–264.

Barrows P (2001) **Kleinian child psychotherapy**. *Clinical Child Psychology and Psychiatry*, in press.

Rustin M, Rhode M, Dubinsky A, *et al* (1997) (eds) **Introduction to Psychotic States in Children**. London: Tavistock/Duckworth.

● CLASSIC PAPERS ●

Henry G (1974) **Doubly deprived**. *Journal of Child Psychotherapy*, **3**, 15–28.

O'Shaughnessy E (1994) **What is a cinical fact?** *International Journal of PsychoAnalysis*, **75**, 939–947.

Shuttleworth J (1998) **Theories of mental development**. *International Journal of Infant Observation*, **1**, 29–50.

● CUTTING EDGE PAPERS ●

Hopkins J (2000) **Overcoming a child's resistance to late adoption: how one new attachment can facilitate another**. *Journal of Child Psychotherapy*, **26**, 335–347.

Orford E (1998) **'Wrestling with the whirlwind': an approach to the understanding of ADD/ADHD**. *Journal of Child Psychotherapy*, **24**, 253–266.

Shuttleworth A (1999) **Finding new clinical pathways in the changing world of district child psychotherapy**. *Journal of Child Psychotherapy*, **25**, 29–49.

Shuttleworth J (1999) **The suffering of Asperger children and the challenge they present to psychoanalytic thinking**. *Journal of Child Psychotherapy*, **25**, 239–265.

● BOOKS ●

Alvarez A (1992) *Live Company*. London: Routledge.

Boston M & Szur R (eds) (1983) *Psychotherapy with Severely Depressive Children*. London: Routledge. Republished by Karnac.

Fonagy P & Roth T (1998) *Therapy with children*. In *What Works for Whom?* London: Guildford Press.

Hurry A (ed.) (1999) *Psychoanalysis and Developmental Therapy*. London: Karnac.

Lanyado M & Horne A (eds) (1999) *Handbook of Child Psychotherapy*. London: Routledge.

Rustin M & Quagliata E (eds) (2000) *Assessment in Child Psychotherapy*. London: Tavistock/ Duckworth.

Tsiantis J (ed.) (2000) *Work with Parents*. London: Karnac.

Waddell M (1998) *Inside Lives: Psychoanalysis and the Growth of the Personality*. London: Tavistock/Duckworth.

MUSIC THERAPY

● SYSTEMATIC REVIEWS AND META-ANALYSES ●

Finkelhor D & Berliner L (1995) **Research on the treatment of sexually abused children: A review and recommendations**. *Journal of the American Academy of Child and Adolescent Psychiatry*, **34**, 1408–1423.

● PAPERS ●

Aasgaard T (2000) **'A Suspiciously Cheerful Lady': a study of a song's life in the paediatric oncology ward, and beyond...** *British Journal of Music Therapy*, **14**, 70–82.

Bruscia K & Stige B (2000) **The nature of meaning in music therapy**. *Nordic Journal of Music Therapy*, **9**, 84–96.

Daveson B A & Kennelly J (2000) **Music therapy in palliative care for hospitalized children and adolescents**. *Journal of Palliative Care*, **16**, 35–38.

Edwards J (1999) **Music therapy with children hospitalised for severe injury or illness**. *British Journal of Music Therapy*, **13**, 21–27.

Tervo J (2001) **Music therapy for adolescents**. *Clinical Child Psychology and Psychiatry*, **6**, 79–91.

● CUTTING EDGE PAPERS ●

Aldridge D, Gustorff D & Neugebauer L (1995) **A preliminary study of creative music therapy in the treatment of children with developmental delay**. *The Arts in Psychotherapy*, **22**, 189–205.

Braithwaite M & Sigafoos J (1998) **Effects of social versus musical antecedents on communication responsiveness in five children with developmental disabilities**. *Journal of Music Therapy*, **35**, 88–104.

Brown S M K (1994) **Autism and music therapy: is change possible, and why music?** *British Journal of Music Therapy*, **8**, 15–25.

Hong M, Hussey D & Heng M (1998) **Music therapy with children with severe emotional disturbances in a residential treatment setting**. *Music Therapy Perspectives*, **16**, 61–66.

Loewy J (2000) **Music psychotherapy assessment**. *Music Therapy Perspectives*, **18**, 47–58.

Montello L & Coons E E (1998) **Effects of active versus passive group music therapy on preadolescents with emotional, learning, and behavioural disorders**. *Journal of Music Therapy*, **35**, 49–67.

Overy, K (2000) **Dyslexia, temporal processing and music: the potential of music as an early learning air for dyslexic children**. *Psychology of Music*, **28**, 218–229.

Robarts J Z (2000) **Music therapy and adolescents with anorexia nervosa**. *Nordic Journal of Music Therapy*, **9**, 3–11.

Robb S L (1996) **Techniques in song writing: restoring emotional and physical well being in adolescents who have been traumatically injured**. *Music Therapy Perspectives*, **14**, 30–37.

—— (2000) **The effect of therapeutic music interventions on the behavior of hospitalized children in isolation: Developing a contextual support model of music therapy**. *Journal of Music Therapy*, **37**, 118–146.

Smeijsters H (1996) **Music therapy with anorexia nervosa: an integrative theoretical and methodological perspective**. *British Journal of Music Therapy*, **10**, 3–13.

Trevarthen C (1999) **Musicality and the intrinsic motive pulse: Evidence from human psychobiology and infant communication**. *Musicae Scientiae*, August, 157–213.

—— & Malloch S N (2000) **The dance of wellbeing: defining the musical therapeutic effect**. *Nordic Journal of Music Therapy*, **9**, 3–17.

Trolldalen G (1997) **Music therapy and interplay: a music therapy project with mothers and children elucidated through the concept of "appreciative recognition"**. *Nordic Journal of Music Therapy*, **6**, 14–27.

Wigram T (2000) **A method of music therapy assessment for the diagnosis of autism and communication disorders in children**. *Music Therapy Perspectives*, **18**, 13–22.

● CLASSIC PAPERS ●

Aldridge D (1989) **A phenomenological comparison of the organisation of music and the self**. *The Arts in Psychotherapy*, **16**, 91–97.

Gaston E T (1968) **Man and music**. In *Music in Therapy* (ed. E Thayer Gaston), pp. 7–29. New York/London: Macmillan.

Sears W W (1968) **Processes in music therapy**. In *Music in Therapy* (ed. E Thayer Gaston), pp. 30–44. New York/London: Macmillan.

● BOOKS ●

Aldridge D (1996) *Music Therapy Research and Practice in Medicine: From Out of the Silence*. London: Jessica Kingsley.

Alvin J & Warwick A (1997) *Music Therapy and the Autistic Child*. Oxford: Oxford University Press.

Bruscia K E (ed.) (1991) *Case Studies in Music Therapy*. Gilsum, NH: Barcelona.

—— (ed.) (1998) *The Dynamics of Music Psychotherapy*. Gilsum, NH: Barcelona.

Bunt L (1994) *Music Therapy: An Art Beyond Words*. London: Routledge.

Hordern P (ed.) (2000) *Music as Medicine. The History of Music Therapy since Antiquity*. Aldershot: Ashgate.

Nordoff P & Robbins C (1971/1998) *Therapy in Music for Handicapped Children*. London: Gollancz.

Pavlicevic M (1997) *Music Therapy in Context: Music, Meaning and Relationship*. London: Jessica Kingsley.

Wigram T & De Backer J (eds) (1999) *Clinical Applications of Music Therapy in Developmental Disability, Paediatrics and Neurology*. London: Jessica Kingsley.

● CD-ROMS AND VIDEOS ●

Aigen K, Turry A & Beer L (1997) *Improvised Song in Group Music Therapy with Adolescents*. Video available in NTSC format from Nordoff-Robbins Center for Music Therapy, New York University. E-mail: Kenneth.Aigen@nyu.edu

Aldridge D (1999) *Music Therapy with Children – CD-ROM*. London: Jessica Kingsley.

Oldfield A (1999) *Music Therapy with Children on the Autistic Spectrum (video)*. Anglia Polytechnic University. Available from British Society for Music Therapy, East Barnet, Herts.

● WEBSITES ●

British Society for Microbiological Technology http://www.bsmt.org.uk

Music Therapy World http://www.musictherapyworld.net

Nordic Journal of Music Therapy http://www.hisf.no/njmt

INTRODUCTION

Until recently, a lack of good quality research meant that pharmacological treatments were considered inappropriate for the majority of children and adolescents suffering from psychiatric disorders. Much of the evidence that was available was from small and often poorly designed studies. However, over the past five years a significant number of larger, often multi-site, studies, with much more rigorous methodologies, have been completed. This has led to drug treatments being increasingly recognised as an appropriate option for children and adolescents, albeit with caution and often in conjunction with psychological treatments.[159] Despite continuing controversy, when used appropriately medication can produce a highly beneficial effect.[160] There remain many unanswered questions, and pharmacological treatments for children and adolescents with psychiatric disorders continue to be inferred from adult studies. There have been few studies that have investigated the pharmacokinetics, pharmacodynamics and safety of psychoactive medications for this patient group, and few psychoactive medications are licensed for use in children and adolescents. This means that pharmacological treatment in the child and adolescent mental health arena rests on the judgement of the individual clinician.[161] The literature in this area continues to grow rapidly and as a result clinical recommendations also change frequently, making this an area of practice where 'keeping up to date' becomes increasingly difficult. Despite these problems, it is clear that developing an understanding of the use of pharmacological treatments is now an essential part of the child and adolescent psychiatrist's training and continuing professional development.

CRITICAL QUESTIONS

by Dr David Coghill

What recent developments have there been in psychopharmacology?

A wealth of new information has been published recently. The National Institute for Mental Health (NIMH) has adopted a strategy of funding large multi-site treatment trials comparing pharmacological and non-pharmacological treatments. The first to be completed and published, the MTA study, has set new standards for clinical trials in our field. One important finding is that the detail of how stimulant medication is titrated and monitored seems to affect its effectiveness. The NIMH has also set up Research Units in Paediatric Psychopharmacology (RUPPs). RUPPs currently consist of a network of seven independent research teams collaborating with the NIMH to conduct high-priority clinical studies into the safety and efficacy of medications for children and adolescents with anxiety disorders, mood disorders and autism.

159   Jacobs B (1993) Treatment in child and adolescent psychiatry. In *Seminars in Child and Adolescent Psychiatry* (eds D Black & D Cottrell), pp. 183–217. London: Gaskell.

160   Taylor E (1994) **Physical treatments**. In *Child and Adolescent Psychiatry: Modern Approaches*. 3rd edn. Oxford: Blackwell Scientific Publications.

161   Medline database.

In view of the failure to demonstrate efficacy of the tricyclic antidepressants (TCAs) in a paediatric population the study of Emslie et al[162] demonstrating the efficacy of fluoxetine in children and adolescents with depression is welcomed; as is the increasing evidence supporting the efficacy and effectiveness, in adult populations, of SSRIs in other emotional and post-traumatic disorders and for the new generation of antipsychotics in schizophrenia. Much of this work now needs replication in the children and adolescent population.

In addition to the many clinical advances, there have also been many major advances in our understanding of the neurobiology of psychiatric disorders. In our field, this has been most relevant with respect to ADHD, where a great deal of effort has gone into linking up basic and clinical science. This is an area in which we can expect to see further major advances in the next few years through methodologies, such as comparative psychopharmacology, across development and across species, pharmacogenomics and functional neuroimaging.

What key messages from new research are not being used?

While caution in the use of psychoactive medication is understandable, and probably desirable, its use often seems idiosyncratic with clinical practice varying widely between individual practitioners. Despite clear evidence to support the effectiveness of pharmacological interventions for ADHD, there is still often a polarised debate over pharmacological v. psychological treatments, and for those receiving medication titration is often haphazard and poorly monitored. The use of non-stimulant medications for which efficacy has been demonstrated, such as buproprion, is rare. It may be that if clinical practice with regard to the use of stimulant medications for ADHD (for which there is a relatively large literature) is unpredictable, then the situation with regard to other classes of drugs and other disorders will be similar if not worse. Lastly, we have yet to see the establishment of large centrally funded and commissioned multi-site research initiatives in the UK to compliment those being carried out under the auspices of the NIMH.

PSYCHOPHARMACOLOGY

● GENERAL PAPERS ●

Riddle M A, Kastelic E A & Frosch E (2001) **Pediatric psychopharmacology**. *Journal of Child Psychology and Psychiatry*, **42**, 73–90.

ATTENTION-DEFICIT HYPERACTIVITY DISORDER

● SYSTEMATIC REVIEWS OR META-ANALYSES ●

Connor D F, Fletcher K E & Swanson J M (1999) **A meta-analysis of clonidine for symptoms of attention-deficit hyperactivity disorder**. *Journal of the American Academy of Child and Adolescent Psychiatry*, **38**, 1551–1559.

Greenhill L, Abikoff H, Arnold E, et al (1996) **Medication treatment strategies in the MTA study: Revelance to clinicians and researchers**. *Journal of the American Academy of Child and Adolescent Psychiatry*, **35**, 1304–1313.

---

162 Emslie G J, Walkup J T, Pliszka S R, et al (1999) **Nontricyclic antidepressants: current trends in children and adolescents**. *Journal of the American Academy of Child & Adolescent Psychiatry*, **38**, 517–528.

Jadad A R, Booker L, Gauld M, *et al* (1999) **The treatment of attention-deficit hyperactivity disorder: an annotated bibliography and critical appraisal of published systematic reviews and meta-analyses**. *Canadian Journal of Psychiatry – Revue Canadienne de Psychiatrie*, **44**, 1025–1035.

——, Boyle M, Cunningham C, *et al* (1999) **Treatment of attention-deficit/ hyperactivity disorder**. Evidence Report. *Technology Assessment* (Summary), **11**, 1–341.

Kavale K (1982). **The efficacy of stimulant drug treatment for hyperactivity: a meta-analysis**. *Journal of Learning Disabilities*, **15**, 280–289.

Klassen A, Miller A, Raina P, *et al* (1999) **Attention-deficit hyperactivity disorder in children and youth: a quantitative systematic review of the efficacy of different management strategies**. *Canadian Journal of Psychiatry – Revue Canadienne de Psychiatrie*, **44**, 1007–1016.

Losier B J, McGrath P J & Klein R M (1996) **Error patterns of the Continuous Performance Test in non-medicated and medicated samples of children with and without ADHD: A meta-analytic review**. *Journal of Child Psychology and Psychiatry and Allied Disciplines*, **37**, 971–987.

Oosterlaan J, Logan G D & Sergeant J A (1998) **Response inhibition in AD/ HD, CD, comorbid AD/HD + CD, anxious, and control children: A meta-analysis of studies with the stop task.** *Journal of Child Psychology and Psychiatry and Allied Disciplines*, **39**, 411–425. (Reviewed on DARE.)

Silva R R, Munoz D M & Alpert M (1996) **Carbamazepine use in children and adolescents with features of attention-deficit hyperactivity disorder: A meta-analysis**. *Journal of the American Academy of Child and Adolescent Psychiatry*, **35**, 352–358.

Stein M A, Krasowski M, Leventhal B L, *et al* (1996) **Behavioral and cognitive effects of methylzanthines: a meta-analysis of theophylline and caffeine**. *Archives of Pediatrics and Adolescent Medicine*, **150**, 284–288.

Thurber S & Walker C E (1983) **Medication and hyperactivity: a meta-analysis**. *Journal of General Psychology*, **108**, 79–86.

● GENERAL PAPERS ●

Pliszka S R, Greenhill L L, Crismon M L, *et al* (2000) **The Texas Children's Medication Algorithm Project: Report of the Texas Consensus Conference Panel on Medication Treatment of Childhood: Attention-Deficit/Hyperactivity Disorder. Part I: Attention-deficit/hyperactivity disorder**. *Journal of the American Academy of Child and Adolescent Psychiatry*, **39**, 908–919.

——, Greenhill L L, Crismon M L, *et al* (2000) **The Texas Children's Medication Algorithm Project: Report of the Texas Consensus Conference Panel on Medication Treatment of Childhood: Attention-Deficit/Hyperactivity Disorder. Part II: Tactics. Attention-deficit/hyperactivity disorder**. *Journal of the American Academy of Child and Adolescent Psychiatry*, **39**, 920–927.

Swanson J M, Cantwell D, Lerner M, *et al* (1993) **Effects of stimulant medication on learning in children with ADHD**. *Exceptional Children*, **60**, 154–161.

Taylor E (1999) **Developmental neuropsychopathology of attention deficit and impulsiveness**. *Development and Psychopathology*, **11**, 607–628.

● CLASSIC PAPERS ●

Bradley C (1937) **The behaviour of children receiving Benzedrine**. *American Journal of Orthopsychiatry*, **15**, 577–585.

● CUTTING EDGE PAPERS ●

Gadow K D, Sverd J, Sprafkin J, *et al* (1999) **Long-term methylphenidate therapy in children with comorbid attention-deficit hyperactivity disorder and chronic multiple tic disorder**. *Archives of General Psychiatry*, **56**, 330–336.

The MTA Cooperative Group Multimodal Treatment Study of Children with ADHD (1999) **A 14-month randomized clinical trial of treatment strategies for attention-deficit/hyperactivity disorder**. *Archives of General Psychiatry*, **56**, 1073–1086.

—— (1999) **Moderators and mediators of treatment response for children with attention-deficit/hyperactivity disorder: the Multimodal Treatment Study of Children with Attention-Deficit/Hyperactivity Disorder**. *Archives of General Psychiatry*, **56**, 1088–1096.

Shader R I, Harmatz J S, Oesterheld J R, *et al* (1999) **Population pharmacokinetics of methylphenidate in children with attention-deficit hyperactivity disorder**. *Journal of Clinical Pharmacology*, **39**, 775–785.

Solanto M V (1998) **Neuropsychopharmacological mechanisms of stimulant drug action in attention-deficit hyperactivity disorder: a review and integration**. *Behavioural Brain Research*, **94**, 127–152.

● REPORTS ●

Gilmore A, Best L & Milne R (1998) *Methylphenidate in Children with Hyperactivity*. DEC Report 78. Bristol: South and West Research and Development Directorate.

Joughin C & Zwi M (1999) *FOCUS on the Use of Stimulants in Children with Attention Deficit Hyperactivity Disorder: A Primary Evidence-Base Briefing*. London: The Royal College of Psychiatrists' Research Unit.

Mental Health Committee, Canadian Paediatric Society (1990) **The use of methylphenidate for attention deficit hyperactivity disorder**. *Canadian Medical Association Journal*, **142**, 817–818.

National Institute of Clinical Excellence (2000) *Guidance on the Use of Methylphenidate (Ritalin, Equasym) for Attention Deficit/Hyperactivity Disorder in Childhood*. Technology Appraisal Guidance – No. 13. London: National Institute of Clinical Excellence.

● BOOKS ●

Solanto M V, Arnsten A F T & Castellanos F X (eds) (2001) *Stimulant Drugs and ADHD, Basic and Clinical Neuroscience*. New York: Oxford University Press.

AUTISM

● REVIEWS ●

Buitelaar J K & Willemsen-Swinkels S H (2000) **Autism: current theories regarding its pathogenesis and implications for rational pharmacotherapy**. *Paediatric Drugs*, **2**, 67–81.

Buitelaar J K & Willemsen-Swinkels S H (2000) **Medication treatment in subjects with autistic spectrum disorders**. *European Child and Adolescent Psychiatry*, **9** (suppl. 1), 85–97.

● CUTTING EDGE PAPERS ●

Campbell M, Anderson L T, Small A M, *et al* (1993) **Naltrexone in autistic children: behavioral symptoms and attentional learning**. *Journal of the American Academy of Child and Adolescent Psychiatry*, **32**, 1283–1291.

McDougle C J, Naylor S T, Cohen D J, *et al* (1996) **A double-blind, placebo-controlled study of fluvoxamine in adults with autistic disorder**. *Archives of General Psychiatry*, **53**, 1001–1008.

——, Scahill L, McCracken J T, *et al* (2000) **Research Units on Pediatric Psychopharmacology (RUPP) Autism Network. Background and rationale for an initial controlled study of risperidone**. *Child and Adolescent Psychiatric Clinics of North America*, **9**, 201–224.

CONDUCT DISORDER

● REVIEWS ●

Malone R P, Delaney M A, Leubbert J F, *et al* (2000) **A double-blind placebo-controlled study of lithium in hospitalized aggressive children and adolescents with conduct disorder**. *Archives of General Psychiatry*, **57**, 649–654.

Stewart J T, Myers W C, Burket R C, *et al* (1990) **A review of the pharmacotherapy of aggression in children and adolescents**. *Journal of the American Academy of Child and Adolescent Psychiatry*, **29**, 269–277.

Zubieta J K & Alessi N E (1993) **Is there a role of serotonin in the disruptive behavior disorders? A literature review**. *Journal of Child and Adolescent Psychopharmacology*, **3**, 11–35.

● CUTTING EDGE PAPERS ●

Findling R L, McNamara N K, *et al* (2000) **A double-blind pilot study of risperidone in the treatment of conduct disorder**. *Journal of the American Academy of Child and Adolescent Psychiatry*, **39**, 509–516.

Klein R G, Abikoff H, Klass E, *et al* (1997) **Clinical efficacy of methylphenidate in conduct disorder with and without attention deficit hyperactivity disorder**. *Archives of General Psychiatry*, **54**, 1073–1080.

EATING DISORDERS

● SYSTEMATIC REVIEWS AND META-ANALYSES ●

Bacaltchuk J & Hay P (1999) **Pharmacotherapy for bulimia nervosa**. Protocol for Cochrane Review. In *The Cochrane Library*, Issue 1. Oxford: Update Software.

● REVIEWS ●

Kotler L A & Walsh B T (2000) **Eating disorders in children and adolescents: pharmacological therapies**. *European Child and Adolescent Psychiatry*, **9** (suppl.), 108–116.

Mitchell J E, Raymond N & Specker S (1993) **A review of the controlled trials of pharmacotherapy and psychotherapy in the treatment of bulimia nervosa**. *International Journal of Eating Disorders*, **14**, 229–247.

● CUTTING EDGE PAPERS ●

Walsh B T, Wilson G T, Loeb K L, *et al* (1997) **Medication and psychotherapy in the treatment of bulimia nervosa**. *American Journal of Psychiatry*, **154**, 523–531.

——, Agras W S, Devlin M J, *et al* (2000) **Fluoxetine for bulimia nervosa following poor response to psychotherapy**. *American Journal of Psychiatry*, **157**, 1332–1334.

● PAPERS ●

Gillberg C & Rastam M (1998) **Drug treatment of adolescent eating disorders**. *International Journal of Psychiatry in Practice*, **2**, 79–82.

Jacobi C (1997) **Comparison of controlled psycho- and pharmacotherapy studies in bulimia and anorexia nervosa**. *Psychotherapy and Psychosomatic Medication and Psychology*, **47**, 346–364.

ELIMINATION DISORDERS

● SYSTEMATIC REVIEWS AND META-ANALYSES ●

Glazener C M & Evans J H (2000) **Tricyclic and related drugs for nocturnal enuresis in children**. Cochrane Review. In *The Cochrane Library*, Issue 4. Oxford: Update Software.

—— & —— (2000) **Desmopressin for nocturnal enuresis in children**. Cochrane Review. In *The Cochrane Library*, Issue 4. Oxford: Update Software.

—— & —— (2000) **Drugs for nocturnal enuresis in children (other than desmopressin and tricyclics)**. Cochrane Review. In *The Cochrane Library*, Issue 4. Oxford: Update Software.

Price K (2000) **What is the role of stimulant laxatives in the management of childhood constipation and soiling?** Protocol for Cochrane Review. In *The Cochrane Library*, Issue 4. Oxford: Update Software.

● CUTTING EDGE PAPERS ●

Sener F, Hasanoglu E & Soylemezoglu O (1998) **Desmopressin versus indomethacin treatment in primary nocturnal enuresis and the role of prostaglandins**. *Urology*, **52**, 878–881.

EMOTIONAL DISORDERS: ANXIETY DISORDER

● SYSTEMATIC REVIEWS AND META-ANALYSES ●

Fawcett J & Barkin R L (1998) **A meta-analysis of eight randomized, double-blind, controlled clinical trials of mirtazapine for the treatment of patients with major depression and symptoms of anxiety**. *Journal of Clinical Psychiatry*, **59**, 123–127.

Gammans R E, Stringfellow J C, Hvizdos A J, *et al* (1992) **Use of busprione in patients with generalized anxiety disorder and coexisting depressive symptoms. A meta-analysis of eight randomized, controlled studies**. *Neuropsychobiology*, **25**, 193–201.

Mendes H A, Lima M S & Hotopf M H (2000) **Serotonin reuptake inhibitors and new generation antidepressants for panic disorder**. Cochrane Review. In *The Cochrane Library*, Issue 4. Oxford: Update Software.

● REVIEWS ●

Allen A J, Leonard H & Swedo S E (1995) **Current knowledge of medications for the treatment of childhood anxiety disorders**. *Journal of the American Academy of Child and Adolescent Psychiatry*, **34**, 976–986.

Velosa J F & Riddle M A (2000) **Pharmacologic treatment of anxiety disorders in children and adolescents**. *Child and Adolescent Psychiatric Clinics of North America*, **9**, 119–133.

● CUTTING EDGE PAPERS ●

Black B & Uhde T W (1994) **Treatment of elective mutism with fluoxetine: a double-blind, placebo-controlled study**. *Journal of the American Academy of Child and Adolescent Psychiatry*, **33**, 1000–1006.

Mancini C, Van Ameringen M, Oakman J M, *et al* (1999) **Serotonergic agents in the treatment of social phobia in children and adolescents: a case series**. *Depression and Anxiety*, **10**, 33–39.

Renaud J, Birmaher B, Wassick S C, *et al* (1999) **Use of selective serotonin reuptake inhibitors for the treatment of childhood panic disorder: a pilot study**. *Journal of Child and Adolescent Psychopharmacology*, **9**, 73–83.

ANXIETY DISORDERS: DEPRESSIVE DISORDER

● SYSTEMATIC REVIEWS AND META-ANALYSES ●

Beasley C M (Jr), Dornseif B E, Bosomworth J C, *et al* (1991) **Fluoxetine and suicide: A meta-analysis of controlled trials for depression**. *British Medical Journal*, **303**, 685–692.

Biederman J, Gonzalez E, Bronstein B, *et al* (1998) **Desipramine and cutaneous reactions in pediatric outpatients**. *Journal of Clinical Psychiatry*, **49**, 178–183.

Churchill R, Wessely S & Lewis G (2000) **Pharmacotherapy and psychotherapy for depression.** Protocol for Cochrane Review. In *The Cochrane Library*, Issue 4. Oxford: Update Software.

Fawcett J & Barkin R L (1998) **A meta-analysis of eight randomized, double-blind, controlled clinical trials of mirtazapine for the treatment of patients with major depression and symptoms of anxiety**. *Journal of Clinical Psychiatry*, **59**, 123–127.

Geller B, Reising D, Leonard H L, *et al* (1999) **Critical review of tricyclic antidepressant use in children and adolescents**. *Journal of the American Academy of Child and Adolescent Psychiatry*, **38**, 513–516.

Hazell P, O'Connell D, Heathcote D, *et al* (1995) **Efficacy of tricyclic drugs in treating child and adolescent depression: a meta-analysis**. *British Medical Journal,* **310**, 897–901.

——, ——, ——, *et al* (2001) **Tricyclic drugs for depression in children and adolescents**. Cochrane Review. In *The Cochrane Library*, Issue 1. Oxford: Update Software.

● CLINICAL GUIDELINES ●

Hughes C W, Emslie G J, Crismon M L, *et al* (1999) **The Texas Children's Medication Algorithm Project: Report of the Texas Consensus Conference Panel on Medication Treatment of Childhood Major Depressive Disorder**. *Journal of the American Academy of Child and Adolescent Psychiatry*, **38**, 1442–1454.

● REVIEWS ●

Ambrosini P J (2000) **A review of pharmacotherapy of major depression in children and adolescents**. *Psychiatric Services*, **51**, 627–633.

Devane C L & Sallee F R (1996) **Serotonin selective reuptake inhibitors in child and adolescent psychopharmacology: a review of published experience**. *Journal of Clinical Psychiatry*, **57**, 55–66.

Emslie G J, Walkup J T, Pliszka S R, *et al* (1999) **Nontricyclic antidepressants: current trends in children and adolescents**. *Journal of the American Academy of Child & Adolescent Psychiatry*, **38**, 517–528.

● CLASSIC PAPERS ●

Puing-Antich J, Perel J M, Lupatkin W, *et al* (1987) **Imipramine in prepubertal major depressive disorders**. *Archives of General Psychiatry*, **44**, 81–89.

● CUTTING EDGE PAPERS ●

Emslie G J, Rush A J, Weinberg W A, *et al* (1997) **A double-blind, randomized, placebo-controlled trial of fluoxetine in children and adolescents with depression**. *Archives of General Psychiatry*, **54**, 1031–1037.

Findling R L, Reed M D, Myers C, *et al* (1999) **Paroxetine pharmacokinetics in depressed children and adolescents**. *Journal of the American Academy of Child and Adolescent Psychiatry*, **38**, 952–959.

Kowatch R A, Carmody T J, Emslie G J, *et al* (1999) **Prediction of response to fluoxetine and placebo in children and adolescents with major depression: a hypothesis generating study**. *Journal of Affective Disorders*, **54**, 269–276.

Reid I C & Stewart C A (2001) **How antidepressants work. New perspectives on the pathophysiology of depressive disorder**. *British Journal of Psychiatry*, **178**, 299–303.

ANXIETY DISORDERS: OBSESSIVE–COMPULSIVE DISORDER

● SYSTEMATIC REVIEWS AND META-ANALYSES ●

Greist J H, Jefferson J W, Kobak K A, *et al* (1995) **Efficacy and tolerability of serotonin transport inhibitors in obsessive–compulsive disorder. A meta-analysis**. *Archives of General Psychiatry*, **52**, 53–60.

Oakley-Browne M & Doughty C (1997) **Psychological and pharmacological treatments of obsessive–compulsive disorder**. Cochrane Review. In *The Cochrane Library*, Issue 1. Oxford: Update Software.

Piccinelli M, Pini S, Bellantuono C, *et al* (1995) **Efficacy of drug treatment in obsessive–compulsive disorder. A meta-analytic review**. *British Journal of Psychiatry,* **166**, 424–434.

Soomro G M, Oakley-Browne M & Doughty C (2000) **Serotonin re-uptake inhibitors (SSRIs) versus placebo for obsessive compulsive disorders**. Protocol for Cochrane Review. In *The Cochrane Library*, Issue 4. Oxford: Update Software.

● REVIEWS ●

Thomsen P H (2000) **Obsessive–compulsive: pharmacological treatment**. *European Child and Adolescent Psychiatry*, **9** (suppl. 1), 76–84.

● CLASSIC PAPERS ●

Leonard H L, Swedo S E, Rapoport J L, *et al* (1989) **Treatment of obsessive–compulsive disorder with clomipramine and desipramine in children and adolescents**. *Archives of General Psychiatry*, **46**, 1088–1092.

● CUTTING EDGE PAPERS ●

de Haan E, Hoogduin K, Buitelaar J, *et al* (1998) **Behavior therapy versus clomipramine in obsessive compulsive disorder in children and adolescence**. *Journal of the American Academy of Child and Adolescent Psychiatry*, **37**, 1022–1029.

March J S, Biederman J, Wolkow R, *et al* (1998) **Sertraline in children and adolescents with obsessive–compulsive disorder: a multicenter randomized controlled trial**. *Journal of the American Medical Association*, **280**, 1752–1756. (Erratum in **283**, 1293.)

McDougle C J, Epperson C N, Pelton G H, *et al* (2000) **A double-blind, placebo-controlled study of risperidone addition in serotonin reuptake inhibitor-refractory obsessive–compulsive disorder**. *Archives of General Psychiatry*, **57**, 794–801.

POST-TRAUMATIC STRESS DISORDER

● SYSTEMATIC REVIEWS AND META-ANALYSES ●

Stein D J, Zungu-Dirwayi N, van der Linden G J H, *et al* (2001) **Pharmacotherapy for posttraumatic stress disorder**. Cochrane Review. In *The Cochrane Library*, Issue 1. Oxford: Update Software.

● REVIEWS ●

Donnelly C L, Amaya-Jackson L & March J S (1999) **Psychopharmacology of pediatric posttraumatic stress disorder**. *Journal of Child and Adolescent Psychopharmacology*, **9**, 203–220.

PSYCHOSIS: MANIA AND BIPOLAR AFFECTIVE DISORDER

● REVIEWS ●

Botteron K N & Geller B (1995) **Pharmacological treatment of childhood and adolescent mania**. *Child and Adolescent Psychiatric Clinics of North America*, **4**, 283–304.

● CUTTING EDGE PAPERS ●

Chang K D & Ketter T A (2000) **Mood stabilizer augmentation with olanzapine in acutely manic children**. *Journal of Child and Adolescent Psychopharmacology*, **10**, 45–49.

Duffy A, Alda M, Kutcher S, *et al* (1998) **Psychiatric symptoms and syndromes among adolescent children of parents with lithium-responsive or lithium-nonresponsive bipolar disorder**. *American Journal of Psychiatry*, **155**, 431–433.

Frazier J A, Meyer M C, Bierderman J, *et al* (1999) **Risperidone treatment for juvenile bipolar disorder: A retrospective chart review**. *Journal of the American Academy of Child and Adolescent Psychiatry*, **38**, 960–965.

Geller B, Cooper T B, Sun K, *et al* (1998) **Double-blind placebo-controlled study of lithium for adolescents with comorbid bipolar and substance dependency**. *Journal of the American Academy of Child and Adolescent Psychiatry*, **37**, 171–178.

——, ——, ——, *et al* (1998) **Lithium for prepubertal depressed children with family history predictors of future bipolarity: a double-blind, placebo-controlled study**. *Journal of Affective Disorders*, **51**, 165–175.

Hagino O R, Weller E B, Weller R A, *et al* (1995) **Untoward effects of lithium treatment in children aged four through six years**. *Journal of the American Academy of Child and Adolescent Psychiatry*, **34**, 1584–1590.

—, —, —, *et al* (1998) **Comparison of lithium dosage methods for preschool- and early school-age children**. *Journal of the American Academy of Child and Adolescent Psychiatry*, **37**, 60–65.

Kowatch R A, Suppes T, Carmody T J, *et al* (2000) **Effect of lithium, divalproex sodium, and carbamazepine in children and adolescents with bipolar disorder**. *Journal of the American Academy of Child and Adolescent Psychiatry*, **39**, 713–720.

PSYCHOSIS: SCHIZOPHRENIA

● SYSTEMATIC REVIEWS AND META-ANALYSES ●

Duggan L, Fenton M, Dardennes R M, *et al* (2001) **Olanzapine for schizophrenia**. Cochrane Review. In *The Cochrane Library*, Issue 1. Oxford: Update Software.

Fenton M, Morris S, DeSilva P, *et al* (2001) **Zotepine for schizophrenia**. Cochrane Review. In *The Cochrane Library*, Issue 1. Oxford: Update Software.

Gilbody S M, Bagnall A M, Duggan L, *et al* (2001) **Risperidone versus other atypical antipsychotic medication for schizophrenia**. Cochrane Review. In *The Cochrane Library*, Issue 1. Oxford: Update Software.

Joy C B, Adams C E & Lawrie S M (1998) **Haloperidol for schizophrenia**. Cochrane Review. In *The Cochrane Library*, Issue 1. Oxford: Update Software.

Srisurapanont M, Disayavanish C & Taimkaew K (1999) **Quetiapine for schizophrenia**. Cochrane Review. In *The Cochrane Library*, Issue 1. Oxford: Update Software.

Tuunainen A, Wahlbeck K & Gilbody S M (2001) **Newer atypical antipsychotic medication versus clozapine for schizophrenia**. Cochrane Review. In *The Cochrane Library*, Issue 1. Oxford: Update Software.

Wahlbeck K, Cheine M & Essali M A (2001) **Clozapine versus typical neuroleptic medication for schizophrenia**. Cochrane Review. In *The Cochrane Library*, Issue 1. Oxford: Update Software.

● REVIEWS ●

Campbell M, Rapoport J L & Simpson G M (1999) **Antipsychotics in children and adolescents**. *Journal of the American Academy of Child and Adolescent Psychiatry*, **38**, 537–545.

Remschmidt H, Hennighausen K, Clement H-W, *et al* (2000) **Atypical neuroleptics in child and adolescent psychiatry**. *European Child and Adolescent Psychiatry*, **9** (suppl.), 9–19.

● CUTTING EDGE PAPERS ●

Kumra S, Frazier J A, Jacobsen L K, *et al* (1996) **Childhood-onset schizophrenia. A double-blind clozapine-haloperidol comparison**. *Archives of General Psychiatry*, **53**, 1090–1097.

● REVIEWS ●

Robertson M M & Strer J S (2000) **Gilles de la Tourette syndrome: Symptomatic treatment based on evidence**. *European Child and Adolescent Psychiatry*, **9** (suppl.), 60–75.

● GENERAL PAPERS ●

Bruun R D & Budman C L (1996) **Risperidone as a treatment for Tourette's syndrome**. *Journal of Clinical Psychiatry*, **57**, 29–31.

Caine E D, Polinsky R J, Kartzinel R, *et al* (1979) **The trial use of clozapine for abnormal involuntary movement disorders**. *American Journal of Psychiatry*, **136**, 317–320.

Chappell P B, Riddle M A, Scahill L, *et al* (1995) **Guanfacine treatment of comorbid attention-deficit hyperactivity disorder and Tourette's syndrome: preliminary clinical experience**. *Journal of the American Academy of Child and Adolescent Psychiatry*, **34**, 1140–1146.

Gilbert D L, Sethuraman G, Sine L, *et al* (2000) **Tourette's syndrome improvement with pergolide in a randomized, double-blind, crossover trial**. *Neurology*, **54**, 1310–1315.

Goetz C G, Tanner C M, Wilson R S, *et al* (1987) **Clonidine and Gilles de la Tourette's syndrome: double-blind study using objective rating methods**. *Annals of Neurology*, **21**, 307–310.

Grothe D R, Calis K A, Jacobsen L, *et al* (2000) **Olanzapine pharmacokinetics in pediatric and adolescent inpatients with childhood-onset schizophrenia**. *Journal of Clinical Psychopharmacology*, **20**, 220–225.

Leckman J F, Hardin M T, Riddle M A, *et al* (1991) **Clonidine treatment of Gilles de la Tourette's syndrome**. *Archives of General Psychiatry*, **48**, 324–328.

Robertson M M, Scull D A, Eapen V, *et al* (1996) **Risperidone in the treatment of Tourette syndrome: a retrospective case note study**. *Journal of Psychopharmacology*, **10**, 317–320.

Sallee F R, Nesbitt L, Jackson C, *et al* (1997) **Relative efficacy of haloperidol and pimozide in children and adolescents with Tourette's disorder**. *American Journal of Psychiatry*, **154**, 1057–1062.

——, Kurlan R, Goetz C G, *et al* (2000) **Ziprasidone treatment of children and adolescents with Tourette's syndrome: a pilot study**. *Journal of the American Academy of Child and Adolescent Psychiatry*, **39**, 292–299.

Singer H S, Brown J, Quaskey S, *et al* (1995) **The treatment of attention-deficit hyperactivity disorder in Tourette's syndrome: a double-blind placebo-controlled study with clonidine and desipramine**. *Pediatrics*, **95**, 74–81.

Section 7: emerging data-sets

Assessment

INTRODUCTION

Assessment in child and adolescent mental health is very complex. The main reasons for the complexity of assessment of children and adolescents are that:

○ concern for a particular problem a child is experiencing is usually explained by a parent (or other adult) on the child's behalf. In fact, the child may not be aware of, or feel that a problem exists;

○ it is important to understand the child's functioning from a variety of sources, for example, school, and interactions between family members; and

○ understanding the developmental stage of the child is important during the assessment process.

A comprehensive assessment of a child or adolescent will include:

○ parents' description of the complaint;

○ history from parents;

○ family interview;

○ interview with the child;

○ physical examination and other observations/investigations; and

○ psychometric testing.[163]

REFERENCES

● PRACTICE PARAMETERS ●

American Academy of Child and Adolescent Psychiatry (1994) **Practice parameters for the assessment and treatment of children and adolescents with schizophrenia**. *Journal of the American Academy of Child and Adolescent Psychiatry*, **33**, 616–635.

—— (1997) **Practice parameters for the assessment and treatment of children and adolescents with bipolar disorder**. *Journal of the American Academy of Child and Adolescent Psychiatry*, **36**, 138–157.

—— (1997) **Practice parameters for the forensic evaluation of children and adolescents who may have been physically or sexually abused**. *Journal of the American Academy of Child and Adolescent Psychiatry*, **36**, 423–442.

---

163 Eminson M (1993) **Assessment in child and adolescent psychiatry**. In *Seminars in Child and Adolescent Psychiatry* (eds D Black & D Cottrell), pp. 75–94. London: Gaskell.

—— (1997) **Practice parameters for the assessment and treatment of children, adolescents and adults with attention deficit hyperactivity disorder**. *Journal of the American Academy of Child and Adolescent Psychiatry*, **36** (suppl.), 85S–121S.

—— (1997) **Practice parameters for the assessment and treatment of children and adolescents with conduct disorder**. *Journal of the American Academy of Child and Adolescent Psychiatry*, **36** (suppl.), 122S–139S.

—— (1998) **Practice parameters for the psychiatric assessment of children and toddlers**. *Abstracts of Clinical Care Guidelines*, **10**, 1–7.

—— (1998) **Practice parameters for the assessment and treatment of children and adolescents with depressive disorders**. *Journal of the American Academy of Child and Adolescent Psychiatry*, **37** (suppl.), 63S–83S.

—— (1998) **Practice parameters for the assessment and treatment of children and adolescents with obsessive–compulsive disorder**. *Journal of the American Academy of Child and Adolescent Psychiatry*, **37** (suppl.), 27S–45S.

—— (1998) **Practice parameters for the assessment and treatment of children and adolescents with posttraumatic stress disorder**. *Journal of the American Academy of Child and Adolescent Psychiatry*, **37** (suppl.), 4S–26S.

—— (1998) **Practice parameters for the assessment and treatment of children and adolescents with language and learning disorders**. *Journal of the American Academy of Child and Adolescent Psychiatry,* **37** (suppl.), 46S–62S.

Sturge C (2001) **Multi-agency approach to assessment**. *Child Psychology and Psychiatry Review*, **6**, 16–20.

● BOOKS ●

Wilkinson I (1998) ***Child and Family Assessment: Cinical Guidelines for Practitioners***. 2nd edn. London: Routledge.

INTRODUCTION

Attachment disorders in childhood refer to a persistent disturbance in a child's ability to interact and relate to others across social situations. An attachment disorder usually begins before the age of five years, and has its roots in a child's earliest relationships with caregivers. It is to be distinguished from autism and pervasive developmental disorders by its uniquely social origins and the child's correspondingly more-or-less normal cognitive functioning.[164]

Attachment disorders are associated with "grossly pathological care" which could include disregard for the child's basic social needs for affection, comfort and stimulation as well as basic physical needs, and the need for a stable primary caregiver leading to a stable child–caregiver attachment.[165] Attachment disorders, which overlap with the developmental concept of disorganized attachments, are commonly linked to unresolved loss and/or trauma experiences in the caregiver, reliably identified by the Adult Attachment Interview.[166]

DIAGNOSIS AND AETIOLOGY

There are two presentations of attachment disorders in the ICD–10 and the DSM–IV–TR classification systems. These are (1) inhibited type (or 'reactive' according to the ICD–10) and (2) disinhibited type.

The inhibited type of attachment disorder refers to a disorder where a child is unable to initiate and respond in a developmentally appropriate way to most social interactions (e.g. having ambivalent responses or being hypervigilant).

A child with a disinhibited type of attachment disorder would show no selection in his or her choice of attachment figures and may include attention-seeking and indiscriminately friendly behaviour.

CRITICAL QUESTIONS

by Dr Howard Steele

What new developments have there been in the past 2–5 years in the management of attachment disorders?

Over the past five years, the presence of attachment disorders (or disorganised attachments) in a range of clinical populations has been confirmed, and the understanding of the aetiological factors underpinning their development has been greatly advanced. The 1999 book edited by Solomon & George[167] brings together the

164 Zeanah C H & Emde R N (1985) Attachment disorders in infancy and childhood. In *Child and Adolescent Psychiatry: Modern Approaches* (eds M Rutter, E Taylor & L Hersov). 3rd edn. Oxford: Blackwell Scientific Publications.

165 American Psychiatric Association (2000) *Diagnostic and Statistical Manual of Mental Disorders*. 4th edn (DSM–IV–TR). Washington DC: APA.

166 Steele H & Steele M (1994) Intergenerational patterns of attachment. In Attachment Processes during Adulthood (eds D Perlman & K Bartholomew), pp. 93–120. (*Advances in Personal Relationships Series*, Vol. 5.) Bristol, PA: Jessica Kingsley Publishers.

167 See Solomon J & George C (1999) *Attachment Disorganization*. New York & London: Guilford Press; Main M & Solomon J (1990) Procedures for identifying infants as disorganized–disoriented during the strange situation. In *Attachment in the Preschool Years: Theory, Research and Intervention* (eds M Greenberg, D Cicchetti & E M Cummings), pp. 121–160. Chicago: University of Chicago Press.

principal findings in one valuable text. In sum, disorganised attachments, observed at 1–2 years in the presence of the caregiver, are signified by fear at the very moment one would expect the distressed child to approach the caregiver. This situation of being deeply afraid of the caregiver who is (presumably) also loved has been described as 'fear without a solution'.[168] For some infants, the persistence of this intolerable state leads to despair and withdrawal, a severe inhibition of attachment behaviour, while for others, a profound exhibition of attachment behaviour results, as if the child is in a frantic search for someone safe to cling to. In the past few years, these two types of reactive attachment disorder have been documented in approximately 40% of those severely neglected institutionalised infants adopted from Romania.[169] These two forms of attachment disorder echo the pioneering observations of 'infants without families'.[170] These profound attachment disturbances, conceptualised as disorganised attachments in the developmental literature, have been observed in infants who fail to thrive, maltreated infants, and infants of chronically mentally ill mothers. An overarching contributing cause of attachment disorganisation is maternal frightening and/or frightened behaviour,[171] which has been shown to be related to unresolved mourning concerning past loss and/or trauma in the mother's experience.[172]

What key messages from new research are not being widely used?

The immense usefulness of developmental research methods including the Adult Attachment Interview and the Ainsworth Strange Situation[173] have yet to be widely applied in clinical settings. Their potential to quickly identify unresolved mourning in parents, and disorganised attachments in infants, should provide immensely valuable opportunities for early intervention and the prevention of long-term mental health problems.[174] Perhaps then clinicians, funding agencies and policy-makers may claim to be living up to John Bowlby's dictum: "A society who values its children, must cherish their parents".

REFERENCES

● SYSTEMATIC REVIEWS AND META-ANALYSES ●

Cowan P A (1997) **Beyond meta-analysis: a plea for a family systems view of attachment**. *Child Development*, **68**, 601–603.

---

168 Solomon J & George C (1999) *Attachment Disorganization*. New York and London: Guilford Press.

169 O'Connor T, Bredenkamp D, Rutter M, *et al* (1999) **Attachment disturbances and disorders in children exposed to early severe deprivation**. *Infant Mental Health Journal*, 20, 10–29.

170 Burlingham D & Freud A (1944) *Infants without Families*. New York: International Universities Press.

171 Lyons-Ruth K & Jacobvitz D (1999) **Attachment disorganization: Unresolved loss, relational violence, and lapses in behavioural and attentional strategies**. In *Handbook of Attachment* (eds J Cassidy & P Shaver), pp. 520–555. New York: Guilford Press.

172 Scheungel C, Bakermans-Kranenburg M J & van Ijzendoorn M H (1999) **Frigentening maternal behaviour linking unresolved loss and disorganized infant attachment**. *Journal of Consulting and Clinical Psychology*, **67**, 54–63.

173 Main M, Kaplan N & Cassidy J (1985) **Security in infancy, childhood and adulthood: A move to the level of representation**. In 'Growing Points in Attachment Theory and Research' (eds I Bretherton & E Waters). *Monographs of the Society for Research in Child Development,* **50**, 66–104; Steele H & Steele M (1994) **Intergenerational patterns of attachment**. In 'Attachment Processes during Adulthood' (eds D Perlman & K Bartholomew). *Advances in Personal Relationships*, **5**, pp. 93–120.

174 Carlson E (1998) **A prospective longitudinal study of attachment disorganization/disorientation**. *Child Development*, **69**, 1107–1128.

van Ijzendoorn M H (1995) **Adult attachment representations, parental responsiveness, and infant attachment: a meta-analysis on the predictive validity of the Adult Attachment Interview**. *Psychological Bulletin,* **117**, 387–403.

—— & Kroonenberg P M (1988) **Cross-cultural patterns of attachment: A meta-analysis of the strange situation**. *Child Development,* **59**, 147–156.

——, Dijkstra J & Bus A G (1995) **Attachment, intelligence, and language: A meta-analysis**. *Social Development,* **4**, 115–128.

——, Juffer F & Duyvesteyn M G C (1996) **Breaking the intergenerational cycle of insecure attachment: a review of the effects of attachment-based interventions on maternal sensitivity and infant security**. *Journal of Child Psychology and Psychiatry and Allied Disciplines,* **36**, 225–248.

——, Marinus H & Bakermans-Kranenburg M J (1996) **Attachment representations in mothers, fathers, adolescents and clinical groups: a meta-analytic search for normative data**. *Journal of Consulting and Clinical Psychology,* **64**, 8–21.

—— & De Wolff M S (1997) **In search of the absent father – meta-analyses of infant–father attachment: a rejoinder to our discussants**. *Child Development,* **68**, 604–609.

Steele H & Steele M (1994) **Intergenerational patterns of attachment**. In *Attachment Processes During Adulthood* (eds D Perlman & K Bartholomew). *Advances in Personal Relationships Series,* **5**, 93–120.

de Wolff M S & van Ijzendoorn M H (1997) **Sensitivity and attachment: a meta-analysis on parental antecedents of infant attachment**. *Child Development,* **68**, 571–591.

● CLASSIC PAPERS ●

Belsky J & Rovine M (1987) **Temperament and attachment security in the strange situation: An empirical rapprochement**. *Child Development,* **58**, 787–795.

Burlingham D & Freud A (1944) **Infants without families**. New York: International Universities Press.

Crockenberg S (1981) **Infant irritability, mother responsiveness, and social support influences on the security of infant–mother attachment**. *Child Development,* **52**, 857–865.

Main M (1990) **Cross-cultural studies of attachment organization: Recent studies, changing methodologies, and the concept of conditional strategies**. *Human Development,* **33**, 48–61.

——, Kaplan N & Cassidy J (1985) **Security in infancy, childhood and adulthood: A move to the level of representation**. In *Growing Points in Attachment Theory and Research* (eds I Bretherton & E Waters), pp. 66–104. *Monographs of the Society for Research in Child Development,* **50**, Serial No. 209.

● CUTTING EDGE PAPERS ●

Carlson E (1998) **A prospective longitudinal study of attachment disorganization/disorientation**. *Child Development,* **69**, 1107–1128.

Fischer-Mamblona H (2000) **On the evolution of attachment disordered behaviour**. *Attachment and Human Development*, **2**, 8–21.

Scheungel C, Bakermans-Kranenburg M J & van Ijzendoorn M H (1999) **Frightening maternal behaviour linking unresolved loss and disorganized infant attachment**. *Journal of Consulting and Clinical Psychology*, **67**, 54–63.

Spangler G & Grossmann K E (1993) **Biobehavioural organization in securely and insecurely attached infants**. *Child Development*, **59**, 1097–1101.

Zeanah C (1996) **Beyond insecurity: a reconceptualisation of attachment disorders in infancy**. *Journal of Consulting and Clinical Psychology*, **64**, 42–52.

● PAPERS ●

Borris N W & Zeanah C H (1999) **Disturbances and disorders of attachment in infancy: An overview**. *Infant Mental Health Journal*, **20**, 1–9.

O'Connor T, Bredenkamp D, Rutter M, *et al* (1999) **Attachment disturbances and disorders in children exposed to early severe deprivation**. *Infant Mental Health Journal*, **20**, 10–29.

West M & George C (1999) **Abuse and violence in intimate adult relationships: New perspectives from attachment theory**. *Attachment and Human Development*, **1**, 137–156.

● BOOKS ●

Belsky J & Cassidy J (1994) **Attachment: theory and evidence**. In *Development Through Life: A Handbook for Clinicians* (eds M Rutter & D Hay), pp. 373–402. Oxford: Blackwell Scientific Publications.

Lieberman A F & Zeanah C H (1999) **Contributions of attachment theory to infant–parent psychotherapy and other interventions with young children**. In *Handbook of Attachment* (eds J Cassidy & P Shaver), pp. 555–574. New York: Guilford Press.

Lyons-Ruth K & Jacobvitz D (1999) **Attachment disorganization: Unresolved loss, relational violence, and lapses in behavioural and attentional strategies**. In *Handbook of Attachment* (eds J Cassidy & P Shaver), pp. 520–555. New York: Guilford Press.

Main M & Solomon J (1990) **Procedures for identifying infants as disorganized-disoriented during the Strange Situation**. In *Attachment in the Preschool Years: Theory, Research and Intervention* (eds M Greenberg, D Cicchetti & E M Cummings), pp. 121–160. Chicago, IL: University of Chicago Press.

Slade A (1999) **Attachment theory and research: Implications for the theory and practice of individual psychotherapy with adults**. In *Handbook of Attachment* (J Cassidy & P Shaver), pp. 575–594. New York: Guilford Press.

Solomon J & George C (1999) *Attachment Disorganization*. New York & London: Guilford Press.

Electroconvulsive therapy

INTRODUCTION

Electroconvulsive therapy (ECT) is the use of electrically induced convulsions as a form of treatment for mental health problems.

The use of ECT use is very rare in the treatment of children and adolescents. ECT is only used in severe cases and where drug treatment has been ineffective.[175] In fact it has been reported that there is insufficient data to recommend ECT as routine treatment for depression in children and adolescents.[176]

REFERENCES

● SYSTEMATIC REVIEWS AND META-ANALYSES ●

Baldwin S & Oxlad M (1996) **Multiple case sampling of ECT administration to 217 minors: review and meta-analysis**. *Journal of Mental Health*, **5**, 451–463.

Rey J M & Walter G (1997) **Half a century of ECT use in young people**. *American Journal of Psychiatry*, **154**, 595–602.

● REVIEWS ●

Bertagnoli M & Borchardt C M (1990) **A review of ECT for children and adolescents**. *Journal of the American Academy of Child and Adolescent Psychiatry*, **29**, 302–307.

● OTHER ●

Duffett R, Hill P & Lelliott P (1999) **Use of electroconvulsive therapy in young people**. *British Journal of Psychiatry*, **175**, 228–230.

---

175 Jacobs B (1993) Treatment in child and adolescent psychiatry. In *Seminars in Child and Adolescent Psychiatry* (eds D Black & D Cottrell), pp. 211–212. London: Gaskell.
    Taylor E (1985) Physical treatments. In *Child and Adolescent Psychiatry: Modern Approaches*. (eds M Rutter, E Taylor & L Hersov). 3rd edn, pp. 890–891. Oxford: Blackwell Scientific Publications.
176 Hazell P (2001) Depression in children and adolescents. In *Clinical Evidence*. Issue 5, 246–252. London: BMJ Publishing Group.

INTRODUCTION

Severe deafness affects a child's ability to understand what is going on around them and their ability to communicate with their family and others. Children with hearing impairments are (approximately three times) more likely to suffer from emotional and behavioural difficulties than the general population.[177]

The causes of mental health difficulties in the hearing-impaired population is possibly a result of disturbed family relationships and inappropriate child-rearing practices/ attitudes.[178]

The treatment of the hearing-impaired child poses several challenges to mental health professionals.

CRITICAL QUESTIONS

by Dr Peter Hindley

What developments have there been in the field of mental health and deafness in the past 2–5 years?

There have been two key areas of development over the past five years. First, in the area of the management of deafness, there is increasing evidence for the effectiveness of a combination of good psychological support to families from the point of diagnosis, the early introduction of sign language and ongoing intervention in the classroom to support social and emotional development.[179]

The second area of development has been in our understanding of the implications of a cultural model of deafness on service development and delivering interventions. It is now clear that we not only need hearing staff with good signing skills but trained deaf staff who can provide linguistic and cultural insight. However, these staff (skilled deaf and hearing) operate far more effectively in specialised services where a 'critical mass' of people come together.[180] A key review paper is Hindley.[181]

What key messages from new research are not currently being used?

Awareness of the effectiveness of the forms of early intervention described above is patchy across the UK but more prevalent in Scandinavia and The Netherlands. Crucially, early psychological support to families and support to develop early communication is often not available. Service providers are beginning to provide specialist training for deaf staff, but this is still extremely limited. Over the next five

---

177 Graham P (1991) *Child Psychiatry: A Developmental Approach*. 2nd edn. Oxford: Oxford University Press.

178 As above.

179 Greenberg M (2000) *Education interventions: prevention and promotion of competence*. In *Mental Health and Deafness* (eds P A Hindley & N Kitson). London: Whurr's.

180 Hindley P A (2000) **Child and adolescent psychiatry**. In *Mental Health and Deafness* (eds P A Hindley & N Kitson). London: Whurr's; Klein H & Kitson N (2000) **Mental health workers: deaf–hearing partnerships**. In *Mental Health and Deafness* (eds P A Hindley & N Kitson). London: Whurr's.

181 Hindley P A (1997) **Research review: psychiatric aspects of hearing impairment**. *Journal of Child Psychology and Psychiatry*, **38**, 101–117.

years, greater emphasis needs to be placed on two areas: evaluating the effectiveness of specialist *v.* generic services; and assessing adaptations to psychological interventions with deaf children and their effectiveness.

REFERENCES

Greenberg M (2000) **Education interventions: prevention and promotion of competence**. In *Mental Health and Deafness* (eds P A Hindley & N Kitson). London: Whurr's.

Hindley P A (1997) **Research review: psychiatric aspects of hearing impairment**. *Journal of Child Psychology and Psychiatry*, **38**, 101–117.

—— (2000) **Child and adolescent psychiatry**. In *Mental Health and Deafness* (eds P A Hindley & N Kitson). London: Whurr's.

Klein H & Kitson N (2000) **Mental health workers: deaf–hearing partnerships**. In *Mental Health and Deafness* (eds P A Hindley & N Kitson). London: Whurr's.

The mental health of children and adolescents from ethnic minorities

INTRODUCTION

Despite an increasing political emphasis on the mental health needs of people from ethnic minorities, research and writing about the specific needs of children and adolescents from ethnic minority groups remains a vastly under-researched area. The recent epidemiological survey from the ONS[182] has included information on the mental health difficulties of children from different ethnic groups. More recent studies have examined the use of mental health services by different ethnic groups,[183] but results of different studies have been contradictory.

While refugee children constitute a small but important subgroup of children and adolescents from ethnic minorities, their needs are often somewhat different from the more settled population.

REFERENCES

● SYSTEMATIC REVIEWS AND META-ANALYSES ●

Chance S E, Kaslow N J, Summerville M B, *et al* (1998) **Suicidal behavior in African American individuals: current status and future directions**. *Cultural Diversity in Mental Health*, **4**, 19–37.

● CLINICAL GUIDELINES ●

None identified.

● REVIEWS ●

Samman R A (2000) **The influence of race, ethnicity and poverty on the mental health of children.** *Journal of Health Care for the Poor and Underserved*, **11**, 100–110.

● REPORTS ●

Hardman E & Harris R (1998) *Developing and Evaluating Community Mental Health Services. Vol. 1: The Bangladeshi Community, Assessment of Need*. London: Tavistock Clinic.

Meltzer H, Gatward R, Goodman R, *et al* (2000) *Mental Health of Children and Adolescents in Great Britain*. London: Office of National Statistics.

Social Services Inspectorate (2000) *Excellence Not Excuses: Inspection of Services for Ethnic Minority Children and Families*. London: Department of Health.

---

182 Meltzer H, Gatward R, Goodman R, *et al* (2000)*The Mental Health of Children and Adolescents in Great Britain*. London: The Stationery Office.
183 e.g. Pumariega A J, Glover S, Holzer C E, *et al* (1998). II. Utilization of mental health services in a tri-ethnic sample of adolescents. *Community Mental Health Journal*, **34**, 145–156.

● PAPERS ●

Bhui K, Christie Y & Bhugra D (1995) **Essential elements in culturally sensitive psychiatric services**. *International Journal of Social Psychiatry*, **41**, 242–256.

Bui K V & Takeuchi D T (1992) **Ethnic minority adolescents and the use of community mental health care services**. *American Journal of Community Psychology,* **20**, 403–417.

Cooper H, Smaje C & Arber S (1998) **Use of health services by children and young people according to ethnicity and social class: secondary analysis of a national survey**. *British Medical Journal*, **317**, 1047–1051.

Goddard N, Subotsky F & Fombonne E (1996) **Ethnicity and adolescent deliberate self-harm**. *Journal of Adolescence*, **19**, 513–521.

Goodman R & Riachards H (1995) **Child and adolescent psychiatric presentations of second generation Afro-Caribbeans in Britain**. *British Journal of Psychiatry*, **167**, 362–369.

Hackett R, Hackett L & Taylor D C (1991) **Psychological disturbance and its associations in the children of the Gujarati community**. *Journal of Child Psychology and Psychiatry*, **32**, 851–856.

Hodes M, Creamer J & Wooley J (1998) **The cultural meanings of ethnic categories**. *Psychiatric Bulletin*, **22**, 20–24.

Kelleher K J, Moore C D, Childs G E, *et al* (1999) **Patient race and ethnicity in primary care management of child behavior problems**. *Medical care*, **37**, 1092–1104.

Kramer T, Evans N & Garralda M E (2000) **Ethnic diversity among child and adolescent psychiatric (CAP) attenders**. *Child Psychology and Psychiatry*, **5**, 169–175.

Pumariega A J, Glover S, Holzer C E, *et al* (1998) **II. Utilization of mental health services in a tri-ethnic sample of adolescents**. *Community Mental Health Journal*, **34**, 145–156.

Rutter M, Yule W, Berger M, *et al* (1974) **Children of West Indian immigrants – I. Rates of behavioural deviance and of psychiatric disorder**. *Journal of Child Psychology and Psychiatry*, **15**, 241–262.

Stern G, Cottrell D & Holmes J (1990) **Patterns of attendance of child psychiatry out-patients with special reference to Asian families**. *British Journal of Psychiatry*, **156**, 384–387.

● BOOKS ●

Bhugra D & Bahl V (eds) (1999) ***Ethnicity: An Agenda for Mental Health***. London: Gaskell.

Dwivedi K N & Varma V P (1996) ***Meeting the Needs of Ethnic Minority Children: A Handbook for Professionals***. London: Jessica Kingsley.

Hopkins A & Bahl V (eds) (1993) ***Access to Health Care for People from Black and Ethnic Minorities***. London: Royal College of Physicians of London.

Littlewood R & Lipsedge M (1997) ***Aliens and Alienists: Ethnic Minorities and Psychiatry***. London: Routledge.

Smaje C (1995) *Health, 'Race' and Ethnicity: Making Sense of the Evidence*. London: King's Fund Institute.

Tizard B & Phoenix A (1993) *Black, White or Mixed Race? Race and Racism in the Lives of Young People of Mixed Parentage*. London: Routledge.

Cochrane Controlled Trials Register
79 hits (keywords: ethnic AND child*)
6 hits (keywords: ethnic minorit* AND child*)

Consultation in child and adolescent mental health services

By Dr Sebastian Kramer

INTRODUCTION

Consultation is a fundamental task in clinical child and adolescent mental health practice. Clinical work often involves complex meetings with groups of various sizes and composition – family, GP, teacher, social worker, etc. Complex cases involve several agencies, and the consultant might be able to identify which others should also be involved either in parallel with or before CAMHS – primary care, paediatric, special education, child protection or youth offending. Consultation skills are also vital because the first consultation may turn out to be the only intervention provided for the referred child or adolescent.

Consultation skills are also important in emergency situations and when dealing with 'frontline' staff.[184] Experienced staff are often quite speedily able to make provisional hypotheses about a case described to them. This is a form of 'triage' also used in Accident and Emergency departments: How serious is this? What kind of intervention is likely to be required, how quickly and by whom?

The efficient use of such encounters can save enormous time and wasted efforts trying to find out about a case by letter or e-mail, or inviting families to clinic appointment when there is very little chance of their attending. Conversation is at the heart of consultation. All senior CAMHS staff must leave time for this crucial work, otherwise they become isolated from the community they serve. The Audit Commission showed that many clinics have dedicated far too little time (less than 2%) for this.[185] Little improvement in the support to tier 1 services can be expected until health authorities make this type of work a requirement in their contracts and service agreements.[185]

● CONSULTATION TO ORGANISATIONS ●

Here the professional work of the staff is the focus, and the idea is to support their reflections on what they do, not to lead or manage change. All child and adolescent psychiatrists in training are expected to provide regular consultations to staff in a child or young person-related agency.[186] There is no pure technique (or pure theory) of staff consultation; it is a hybrid of training, teaching and therapy, in varying proportions.

---

184 Richardson G & Partridge I (2000) **Child and adolescent mental health service liaison with tier 1 services.** *Psychiatric Bulletin*, **24**, 462–463.

185 Audit Commission (1999) *Children in Mind*. London: Audit Commission.

186 From the *Advisory Papers* of the Child and Adolescent Psychiatry Specialist Advisory Sub-Committee (CAPSAC) of the Royal College of Psychiatrists, November 1999.

REFERENCES

● REVIEWS ●

Steinberg D (1992) **Informed consent: consultation as a basis for collaboration between disciplines and between professionals and their patients.** *Journal of Interprofessional Care*, **6**, 43–48.

—— (1993) **Consultative work in child and adolescent psychiatry.** In *Managing Children with Psychiatric Problems* (ed. M E Garralda), pp. 115–125. London: British Medical Journal Publishing Group.

—— (2000) **The child psychiatrist as consultant to schools and colleges**. In *New Oxford Textbook of Psychiatry* (eds M Gelder, J J Lopez-Ibor & N Andreason), Vol. 2, pp. 1923–1928. Oxford: Oxford University Press.

—— & Yule W (1985) **Consultative work**. In *Child and Adolescent Psychiatry: Modern Approaches* (eds M Rutter & L Hersov), pp. 914–926. 2nd edn. Oxford: Blackwell Scientific Publications.

● CLASSIC PAPERS ●

Menzies I E P (1988) *Selected Essays: Containing Anxiety in Institutions*. London: Free Association's Books.

● BOOKS ●

Caplan G (1970) *The Theory and Practice of Mental Health Consultation*. London: Tavistock.

Gallesich J (1982) *The Profession and Practice of Consultation: A Handbook for Consultants, Trainers of Consultants and Consumers of Consultation Services*. London: Jossey-Bass.

Schlapobersky J R (ed.) (1991) *Institutes and How to Survive Them. Mental Health Training and Consultation*. London: Routledge. (Selected papers by Robin Skynner.)

Steinberg D (1989) *Interprofessional Consultation: Innovation and Imagination in Working Relationships*. Oxford: Blackwell Scientific Publications.

—— (2000) *Letters from the Clinic. Letter Writing in Clinical Practise for Mental Health Professionals*. London: Routledge.

—— (2000) **The child psychiatrists as consultant to schools and colleges**. In *New Oxford Textbook of Psychiatry* (eds M Gelder, J J Lopez-Ibor & N Andreasen), Vol. 2, pp. 1923–1928. Oxford: Oxford University Press.

CRITICAL QUESTIONS

by Mr Anthony Harbour

What important new developments have there been in the law in the past 2–5 years?

One of the most significant legal developments in this area was the implementation of the Human Rights Act 1998 in October 2000. The Human Rights Act incorporates the European Convention of Human Rights into UK law. The most significant Convention Articles for practitioners in this area will be Article 6, the Right to a Fair Trial, and Article 8, the Right to Respect for Private and Family Life.

What key messages from new law are not being fully understood in clinical practice?

The impact of the implementation of the Act, incorporating the European Convention on Human Rights into UK law, is not yet fully understood. Practitioners in this area need to understand the law and be alert to the areas of possible impact on their practice.

REFERENCES

● CASE LAW ●

This is not an exhaustive list of case law in this area. The law reports referenced will all contain a list of cases referred to in the particular judgement that will provide a starting point for identifying other cases that are relevant to the issues in question. The British Medical Association's *Consent, Rights and Choices in Health Care for Children and Young People* (2001) contains comprehensive references to most of the cases involving children in this area.

Gillick *v.* West Norfolk and Wisbech Area Health Authority and another [1986] 1 FLR 224.

Nielsen *v.* Denmark [1988] 11 EHRR 175.

Re R (A Minor) (Wardship: Medical Treatment) [1992] Fam 11 [1991] 4, All ER, 177.

Re W (A minor) 1993 1 FLR 1.

Re W (A minor) (Medical Treatment: Court's jurisdiction) [1993] FAM 64.

Re E (A minor) (Wardship: Medical Treatment) [1991] 2 FLR 585.

South Glamorgan CC *v.* W & B [1993] 1 FLR 574.

R *v.* Kirklees MBC ex parte C [1993] 2FLR 187.

Re K, W and H (minors) (Medical Treatment) [1993] 1FLR 854.

Northampton HA *v.* Official Solicitor and Governors of St Andrews [1994] 1FLR 162.

Re C (Detention: Medical Treatment) [1997] 2 FLR 1980.

Re C (A child) (HIV testing) [1999] 2 FLR 1004.

Re M [1999] 2 FLR 1097.

Sidway *v.* Bethlem Royal Hospital Governors and others [1985] 1 All ER 643.

● GUIDELINES ●

Alderson P & Montgomery J (1996) *Health Care Choices Making Decisions with Children*. London: Institute of Public Policy Research.

British Medical Association and The Law Society (1995) *Assessment of Mental Capacity*. London: BMA.

General Medical Council (1999) *Seeking Patient's Consent: The Ethical Considerations*. London: GMC.

Shaw M (1999) *Treatment Decisions in Young People: The Legal Framework*. London: FOCUS, The Royal College of Psychiatrists' Research Unit.

—— (1999) *Treatment Decisions in Young People: Clinical Guidelines*. London: FOCUS, The Royal College of Psychiatrists' Research Unit.

—— (1999) *Treatment Decisions in Young People: Frequently Asked Questions and References*. London: FOCUS, The Royal College of Psychiatrists' Research Unit.

● CLASSIC PAPERS ●

Bates P (1994) **Children in secure psychiatric units: Re K, Wand H – "out of sight, out of mind?"** *Child Law*, **6**.

Pearce J (1994) **Consent to treatment during childhood: the assessment of competence and avoidance of conflict**. *British Journal of Psychiatry*, **165**, 713–716.

Roth L, Meisel A & Lidz C (1977) **Tests of competence to consent to treatment**. *American Journal of Psychiatry*, **134**, 279.

Rylance G, Bowen C & Rylance J (1995) **Measles and rubella immunisation: information and consent in children**. *British Medical Journal*, **311**, 923–924.

Shaw A (1973) **Dilemmas of 'informed consent' in children**. *The New England Journal of Medicine*, **289**, 885–890.

Weithorn L A & Campbell S B (1982) **The competency of children and adolescents to make informed treatment decisions**. *Child Development*, **53**, 1589–1599.

● BOOKS ●

Alderson P (1993) *Children's Consent to Surgery*. Buckingham: Open University Press.

Black D, Harris-Hendriks J & Woolkind S (eds) *Child Psychiatry and the Law*. 3rd edn. London: Gaskell.

British Medical Association (2001) *Consent, Rights and Choices in Health Care for Children and Young People*. London: BMA.

Cordess C, Bailey S, Trowell J, *et al* (2001) *Confidentiality and Mental Health*. London: Jessica Kingsley.

Kennedy I & Grubb A (2000) *Medical Law*. 3rd edn. Butterworths: London.

Harper R & Butler-Sloss E (1999) *Medical Treatment and the Law*. Bristol: Jordan Publishing.

NHS Health Advisory Service (1995) **Young people, mental health and the law**. In *Child and Adolescent Mental Health Services: Together we stand*. Annex A, pp. 167–182. London: HMSO.

Swindells H, Neaves A, Kushner M, *et al* (1999) **Family law and the Human Rights Act 1998**. Bristol: Jordan Publishing.

Williams R & White R (1996) *Safeguards for Young Minds*. London: Gaskell.

● FOCUS REPORTS ●

Shaw M (1999) *Treatment Decisions in Young People: the Legal Framework*. London: FOCUS, The Royal College of Psychiatrists' Research Unit.

—— (1999) *Treatment Decisions in Young People: Clinical Guidelines*. London: FOCUS, The Royal College of Psychiatrists' Research Unit.

—— (1999) *Treatment Decisions in Young People: Frequently Asked Questions and References*. London: FOCUS, The Royal College of Psychiatrists' Research Unit.

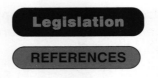

REFERENCES

● **PRACTITIONERS' TEXTBOOKS** ●

The Family Court Practice (2001) *Family Law*. Bristol: Jordan Publishing.

Munro P & Forrester L (1999) *The Guardian ad Litem: Law and Practice*. 2nd edn. Bristol: Jordans.

White R, Carr P & Lowe N (1995) *The Children Act in Practice*. London: Butterworths.

● **GUIDANCE ISSUED BY THE DEPARTMENT OF HEALTH** ●

Department of Health (1990) *An Introduction to the Children Act 1989*. London: HMSO.

—— (1990) *The Care of Children – Principles and Practice in Regulations and Guidance*. London: HMSO.

—— (1991) *Court Orders* (grey book). Children Act 1989 Guidance and Regulations, vol. 1. London: HMSO.

—— (1991) *Family Placements* (orange book). Children Act 1989 Guidance and Regulations, vol. 3. London: HMSO.

—— (1991) *Family Support, Day Care and Educational Provision for Young Children* (blue book). Children Act 1989 Guidance and Regulations, vol. 2. London: HMSO.

—— (1991) *Residential Care* (yellow book). Children Act 1989 Guidance and Regulations, vol. 4. London: HMSO.

—— (1991) *Working Together*. London: HMSO.

——, Home Office & Department for Education and Employment (1999) *Working Together to Safeguard Children*. London: The Stationery Office.

● **ESSENTIAL DEPARTMENT OF HEALTH PUBLICATIONS** ●

Department of Health (1985) *Social Work Decisions in Child Care – Recent Research Findings and their Implications*. London: HMSO.

—— (1988) *Protecting Children – A Guide for Social Workers Undertaking a Comprehensive Assessment*. London: HMSO.

—— (1989) *A Guide for Guardians ad Litem in Public Law Proceedings under the Children Act 1989*. London: Department of Health.

—— (1991) *Patterns and Outcomes and Child Placement: Messages from Current Research and their Implications*. London: HMSO.

—— (1993) *Memorandum of Good Practice: A Guide on Interviewing*. London: HMSO.

—— (1995) *The Challenge of Partnership in Child Protection: Practice Guide*. London: HMSO.

—— (1995) *Child Protection: Messages from Research*. London: HMSO.

—— (1996) *Avoiding Delay in Children Act Cases*. London: HMSO.

—— (1996) *Reporting to Court under the Children Act*. London: HMSO.

—— (1999) *Framework for the Assessment of Children in Need and their Families*. London: The Stationery Office.

● RECOMMENDED READING ●

Adock M & White R (1998) *Significant Harm: its Management and Outcome*. Croydon: Significant Publications.

Children Act Advisory Committee (1997) *Children Act Advisory Committee Report (1996/1997)*. London: Lord Chancellor's Department, Family Policy Division.

Hunt J & Macleod A (1998) *Statutory Intervention in Child Protection*. Bristol: University of Bristol. (Note: this is a thematic summary of two reports entitled *The Last Resort, Child Protection, the Courts and the 1989 Act* and *Parental Perspectives on Care Proceedings.*)

King P & Young I (1992) *The Child as a Client: A Handbook for Solicitors Who Represent Children*. Bristol: Jordan Publishing.

Lindley B (1994) **On the Receiving End: families experiences of the court process in care and supervision proceedings under the Children Act 1989.** London: Family Rights Group.

Wilson K & James A (eds) (1995) *The Child Protection Handbook*. London: Baillière-Tindall.

● BRITISH AGENCIES FOR ADOPTION AND FOSTERING PUBLICATIONS ●

Address: Skyline House, 200 Union Street, London SE1 0LX. Tel: 020 7593 2072.

Batty D (1991) *Sexually Abused Children – Making Placements Work*. London: British Agencies for Adoption and Fostering.

—— (1993) *HIV Infection and Children in Need*. London: British Agencies for Adoption and Fostering.

—— & Cullen D (1996) *Child Protection. The Therapeutic Option*. London: British Agencies for Adoption and Fostering.

Chennells P & Hammond C (1998) *Adopting a Child*. London: British Agencies for Adoption and Fostering.

—— & Morrison M (1998) *Talking About Adoption*. London: British Agencies for Adoption and Fostering.

Falberg V (1994) *A Child's Journey Through Placement*. London: British Agencies for Adoption and Fostering.

Fratter J, Rowe J, Sapsford D, *et al* (1991) *Permanent Family Placement*. London: British Agencies for Adoption and Fostering.

Phillips R & McWilliam E (1996) *After Adoption. Working with Adoptive Families*. London: British Agencies for Adoption and Fostering.

Rushton A, Treseder J & Quinton D (1988) *New Parents for Older Children*. London: British Agencies for Adoption and Fostering.

● RECOMMENDED PERIODICALS ●

Adoption and Fostering London   British Agency for Adoption and Fostering, Skyline House, 200 Union Street, London SE1 0LX.

Child and Family Law Quarterly   Jordan and Sons, 21 St Thomas Street, Bristol BS1 6JS.

Childright   Children's Legal Centre, PO Box 3314, London N1 2WA.

Family Law   Jordan and Sons, 21 St Thomas Street, Bristol BS1 6JS.

Representing Children   National Youth Advocacy Service, quarterly journal: 1 Dawnham Road South, Heswell, Wirral, CH60 5RG.

Seen and Heard   National Association of Guardians *ad litem* and Reporting Officers (NAGALR), 1 Dawnham Road South, Heswell, Wirral, CH60 5RG.

Parenting assessment

INTRODUCTION

Parenting assessments in child care court cases under the 1989 Children Act are primarily an issue of clinical skills guided by theoretical principles and research literature.

The commonly accepted theoretical framework describes parenting as a relationship that is affected by factors in the parents (especially their personalities and own experiences of being parented), in the child (e.g. vulnerability or resilience), and in their living circumstances (e.g. poverty, isolation, or the couple's relationship). In practice, a distinction needs to be made between family assessments in everyday clinical practice (e.g. as part of a behavioural parenting intervention), assessments by social workers and guardians *ad litem* in court proceedings, professional opinions by mental health professionals (based on their previous or current clinical involvement with the family) and independent expert opinions by mental health professionals mandated by the court.

Expert parenting assessments address all aspects of the parent–child relationship that impact on the child's welfare and therefore are more inclusive than risk assessments (of child maltreatment).

CRITICAL QUESTIONS

by Dr Peter Reder

What developments have there been in the field of parenting assessment in the past 2–5 years?

The Department of Health[187] has published guidance for social workers on assessment of children in need and their families, which includes the need for cooperation from mental health services and the use of certain structured assessment techniques to augment clinical interviews. Research and clinical initiatives have guided assessments by focusing attention on the impact of parental mental health problems and domestic violence on children's welfare, the validity of children's accounts of their parenting experiences, and recognition of maltreatment through neglect and illness induction.

What are the key messages from new research that are not being widely used?

Parenting assessments must prioritise the child's welfare and how the parent–child relationship is experienced from the child's perspective. If the parent has a psychiatric disorder, the prognosis of his or her disorder is only one element of a much wider assessment – opinions about parenting capacity should never be based solely on this one factor. Traditional psychological tests, devised to measure intelligence and personality, were not designed to evaluate an adult's capacity to care for children. They only bear an indirect relationship to parenting capacity and research has not yet examined their ability to predict parenting effectiveness. Hence, opinions about parenting should not be over-reliant on such findings.

---

187 Department of Health, Department for Education and Employment & The Home Office (2000) *Framework of the Assessment of Children in Need and their Families*. London: The Stationery Office.

REFERENCES

● REVIEWS ●

Bentovim A (1998) **Significant harm in context**. In *Significant Harm: Its Management and Outcome* (eds M Adcock & R White), pp. 153–202. 2nd edn. Croydon: Significant Publications.

Budd K S & Holdsworth M J (1996) **Issues in the clinical assessment of minimal parenting competence**. *Journal of Clinical Child Psychology*, **25**, 2–14.

Gopfert M, Webster J, Pollard J, *et al* (1996) **The assessment and prediction of parenting capacity: a community-oriented approach**. In *Parental Psychiatric Disorder: Distressed Parents and their Families* (eds M Gopfert, J Webster & M V Seeman), pp. 271–309. Cambridge: Cambridge University Press.

Mrazek D A, Mrazek P & Klinnert M (1995) *Clinical assessment of parenting*. *Journal of the American Academy of Child and Adolescent Psychiatry*, **34**, 272–282.

● CLINICAL GUIDELINES ●

Drummond D C & Fitzpatrick G (2000) **Children of substance misusing parents**. In *Family Matters: Interfaces between Child and Adult Mental Health* (eds P Reder, M McClure & A Jolley), pp. 135–149. London: Routledge.

Glaser D (1993) **Emotional abuse**. In *Clinical Pediatrics: International Practice and Research* (eds J C Hobbs & J M Wynne). London: Baillière Tindall.

Henry L A & Kumar R C (1999) **Risk assessments of infants born to parents with a mental health problem or a learning disability**. In *Child Protection and Adult Mental Health: Conflict of Interest?* (eds A Weir & A Douglas), pp. 49–62. Oxford: Butterworth-Heinemann.

Iwaniec D (1995) **Assessing emotional abuse and neglect**. In *The Emotionally Abused and Neglected Child: Identification, Assessment and Intervention*, pp. 83–100. Chichester: John Wiley and Sons.

Jacobsen T, Miller L J & Kirkwood K (1997) **Assessing parenting competence in individuals with severe mental illness: A comprehensive service**. *Journal of Mental Health Administration*, **24**, 189–199.

Jenner S (1997) **Assessment of parenting in the context of child protection using the parent/child game**. *Child Psychology and Psychiatry Review*, **2**, 58–62.

Milner J S (1994) **Assessing physical child abuse risk: The Child Abuse Potential Inventory**. *Clinical Psychology Review*, **14**, 547–583.

Swadi H (1994) **Parenting capacity and substance misuse: An assessment scheme**. *ACPP Review and Newsletter*, **16**, 237–244.

● CLASSIC PAPERS ●

Kelmer-Pringle M (1978) **The needs of children.** In *The Maltreatment of Children* (ed. S M Smith), pp. 221–243. Lancaster: MTP Press.

Rutter M & Quinton D (1984) **Parental psychiatric disorder: effects on children**. *Psychological Medicine*, **14**, 853–880.

● CUTTING EDGE PAPERS ●

Reder P & Duncan S (1999) **Unresolved conflicts**. In *Lost Innocents: A Follow-up Study of Fatal Child Abuse*, pp. 62–81. London Routledge.

Wilkinson I (2000) **The Darlington family assessment system: Clinical guidelines for practitioner**. *Journal of Family Therapy*, **22**, 211–224.

● BOOKS ●

Belsky J & Vondra J (1989) **Lessons from child abuse: The determinants of parenting**. In *Child Maltreatment: Theory and Research on the Causes and Consequences of Child Abuse and Neglect* (eds D Cicchetti & V Carlson), pp. 153–202. Cambridge: Cambridge University Press.

Department of Health, Cox A & Bentovim A (2000) *Framework for the Assessment of Children in Need and Their Families: The Family Assessment Pack of Questionnaires and Scales*. London: The Stationery Office.

Department of Health, Department of Education and Employment & Home Office (2000) *Framework for the Assessment of Children in Need and Their Families*. London: The Stationery Office.

Herbert M (1996) *Assessing Children in Need and Their Parents*. Leicester: British Psychological Society Books.

Reder P & Lucey C (eds) (1995) *Assessment of Parenting: Psychiatric and Psychological Contributions*. London: Routledge.

INTRODUCTION

● PREVENTION AND HEALTH EDUCATION ●

Prevention and health education programmes appear to be more effective in modifying knowledge, attitudes and normative beliefs rather than changing behaviour. Also, in practice, prevention and health education intentions are frequently undermined by conflicting paradigms that vie for legitimacy (and funding) – a moral approach based on abstinence, and a psychosocial approach that aims to increase knowledge and skills and build social competence.

● MENTAL HEALTH PROMOTION ●

Mental health promotion focuses on public awareness and understandings about mental health to encourage the earlier recognition of the signs of emotional and psychological distress and add to knowledge about the help available (including appropriate self-help). Effective initiatives motivate families and young people to seek help at an early stage and can increase their participation and concordance with treatment.

Ideally, mental health promotion initiatives emphasise holistic approaches that respect local cultures and beliefs, and the need to promote both positive health and ill-health prevention.

● NEEDS ASSESSMENT ●

The appropriate assessment of need for prevention, education and mental health promotion is essential.

One of the factors that may influence prevention and education programmes is that the low base rate of many child and adolescent disorders makes it difficult to see the explicit effects of any intervention programme. Also, socio-economic, cultural and age-related factors affect how people perceive mental health and mental illness. Thus, mental health promotion should be built around prior assessments of existing attitudes and beliefs, and accompanied by appropriate evaluation.

CRITICAL QUESTIONS

by Ms Helen Shaw

What key messages from new research are not being used in the field?

Many mental health promotion initiatives lack impact because they are not based on sound health promotion principles. The latter emphasise holistic culturally sensitive approaches and participatory methods, and where necessary, stress the need to work structurally to address the barriers that exist to mental health and well-being.[188]

Greater use of cost–benefit analysis in programme evaluation can identify the programmes that offer the best social investment. Agencies can also use cost-effectiveness

---

188   Secker J, Armstrong C & Hill M (1999) **Young people's understanding of mental illness.** *Health Education Research*, **14**, 729–739.

analysis to make the best use of their resources, and providers should include cost analysis components in designing their prevention programmes. This can provide greater clarity of the programme goals and objectives and better define the parameters for analysing effectiveness.

REFERENCES

● SYSTEMATIC REVIEWS AND META-ANALYSES ●

Davis M K & Gidycz C A (2000) **Child sexual abuse prevention programs: a meta-analysis**. *Journal of Clinical Child Psychology*, **29**, 257–265.

Durlak J A & Wells A M (1997) **Primary prevention mental health programs for children and adolescents: a meta-analytic review**. *American Journal of Community Psychology*, **25**, 115–152. (Reviewed on DARE.)

—— & —— (1998) **Evaluation of indicated preventative intervention (secondary prevention) mental health programs for children and adolescents**. *American Journal for Community Psychology*, **26**, 775–802. (Reviewed on DARE.)

Harrington R, Whittacker J & Shoebridge P (1998) **Psychological treatment of depression in children and adolescents: A review of treatment research**. *British Journal of Psychiatry*, **173**, 291–298. (Reviewed on DARE.)

Hodnett E D & Roberts I (1999) **Home-based social support for socially disadvantaged mothers**. Cochrane Review. In *The Cochrane Library*, Issue 4. Oxford: Update Software.

Joiner T E J & Wagner K D (1996) **Parental, child-centered attributions and outcome: A meta-analytic review with conceptual and methodological implications**. *Journal of Abnormal Child Psychology*, **24**, 37–52.

Kibby M Y, Tyc V L & Mulhern R K (1998) **Effectiveness of psychological intervention for children and adolescents with chronic medical illness: a meta-analysis**. *Clinical Psychology Review*, **18**, 103–117.

Kok G, van den Borne B & Mullen P D (1997) **Effectiveness of health education and health promotion: meta-analyses of effect studies and determinants of effectiveness**. *Patient Education and Counselling*, **30**, 19–27.

Kolbe L J (1997) **Meta-analysis of interventions to prevent mental health problems among youth: a public health commentary**. *American Journal of Community Psychology*, **25**, 227–232.

Lapalme M, Hodgins S & La Roche C (1997) **Children of parents with bipolar disorder: a metaanalysis of risk for mental disorders**. *Canadian Journal of Psychiatry*, **42**, 623–631.

NHS Centre for Reviews and Dissemination (1997) ***Mental Health Promotion in High Risk Groups***. York: NHS Centre for Reviews and Dissemination. (Reviewed in the Cochrane Library.)

Nicholas B & Broadstock M (1999) ***Effectiveness of Early Interventions for Preventing Mental Illness in Young People: A Critical Appraisal of the Literature***. New Zealand Health Technology Assessment (NZHTA) 1877235113. Christchurch: New Zealand Health Technology Assessment. (Reviewed in the Cochrane Library.)

Ploeg J, Ciliska D, Dobbins M, *et al* (1995) ***A Systematic Overview of the Effectiveness of Public Health Nursing Interventions: An Overview of***

Adolescent Suicide Prevention Programs, pp. 48. University of Toronto, McMaster University: Quality of Nursing Worklife Research Unit. (Reviewed on DARE.)

Reid W J & Crisafulli A (1990) **Marital discord and child behavior problems: a meta-analysis**. *Journal of Abnormal Child Psychology*, **18**, 105–117.

Rispens J, Aleman A & Goudena P P (1997) **Prevention of child abuse victimization: A meta-analysis of school programs**. *Child Abuse and Neglect*, **21**, 975–987. (Reviewed on DARE.)

Sussman S, Lichtman K, Ritt A, *et al* (1999) **Effects of thirty-four adolescent tobacco use cessation and prevention trials on regular users of tobacco products**. *Substance Use and Misuse*, **34**, 1469–1503. (Reviewed on DARE.)

Tobler N S, Roona M R, Ochshorn P, *et al* (2000) **School-based adolescent drug prevention programs: 1998 meta-analysis**. *Journal of Primary Prevention*, **20**, 275–336.

Weissberg R P & Bell D N (1997) **A meta-analytic review of primary prevention programs for children and adolescents: contributions and caveats**. *American Journal of Community Psychol*ogy, **25**, 207–214.

Zoritch B & Roberts I (1999) **Day care for pre-school children**. Cochrane Review. In *The Cochrane Library*, Issue 1. Oxford: Update Software.

● CLINICAL GUIDELINES ●

Arthur B, Elster M D & Kuznets N J (1997) **Guidelines for Adolescent Preventive Services (GAPS)**. *Archives of Pediatric Adolescent Medicine*, **151**, 123–128.

● REVIEWS ●

Gilvarry E (2000) **Substance abuse in young people**. *Journal of Child Psychology and Psychiatry*, **41**, 55–80.

Jensen B B (1997) **A case of two paradigms within health education**. *Health Education Research*, **12**, 419–428.

Mellanby A R, Rees J B & Tripp J H (2000) **Peer-led and adult-led school health education: a critical review of available comparative research**. *Health Education Research*, **15**, 533–545.

Parkin S & McKeganey N (2000) **The rise and rise of peer education approaches**. *Drugs: education, prevention and policy*, **7**, 293–310.

Resnick M D (2000) **Protective factors, resiliency and healthy youth development**. *Adolescent Medicine*, **11**, 157–165.

Seeker J (1998) **Current conceptualisations of mental health and mental health promotion**. *Health Education Research*, **13**, 57–66.

● CLASSIC PAPERS ●

Resnick M D, Harris L J & Blum R W (1993) **The impact of caring and connectedness on adolescent health and well-being.** *Journal of Paediatrics and Child Health*, **29** (suppl.), S3–S9.

Rutter M (1985) **Resilience in the face of adversity: protective factors and resistance to psychiatric disorder**. *British Journal of Psychiatry*, **147**, 598– 611.

—— (1993) **Resilience: some conceptual considerations.** *Journal of Adolescent Health*, **14**, 626–639.

● CUTTING EDGE PAPERS ●

Boys A, Marsden J, Fountain J, *et al* (1999) **What influences young people's use of drugs? A qualitative study of decision-making**. *Drugs: education, prevention and policy*, **6**, 373–387.

Goldston S E (1998) **Cost analysis and primary prevention: a sound idea whose time has come**. *Journal of Mental Health*, **7**, 505–518.

Jorm A F (2000) **Mental health literacy: public knowledge and beliefs about mental disorders**. *British Journal of Psychiatry*, **177**, 396–401.

● REPORTS ●

Hansen W B & McNeal R B (1999) **Drug education practice: results of an observational study**. *Health Education Research*, **14**, 85–87.

Jorm A F, Korten A E, Jacomb P A, *et al* (1997) **Helpfulness of interventions for mental disorders: beliefs of health professionals compared with the general public**. *British Journal of Psychiatry*, **171**, 233–237.

Moore A & Gray A M (eds) (1995) **Evidence-based prevention**, *Bandolier*, October, 20–23.

Nastasi B K (1998) **A model for mental health programming in schools and communities: introduction to the mini-series**. *School Psychology Review*, **27**, 165–174.

Neumark-Sztainer D, Story M, French S A, *et al* (1997) **Psychosocial correlates of health compromising behaviours among adolescents**. *Health Education Research*, **12**, 37–52.

Pavis S, Masters H & Cunningham-Burley S (1996) *Lay Concepts of Mental Health and How it can be Maintained*. Edinburgh: Department of Public Health Sciences, University of Edinburgh.

Paykel E S, Hart D & Priest R G (1998) **Changes in public attitudes to depression during the Defeat Depression Campaign**. *British Journal of Psychiatry*, **173**, 519–522.

Resnick M D, Bearman P S, Blum R W, *et al* (1997) **Protecting adolescents from harm: findings from the national longitudinal study on adolescent health**. *Journal of the American Medical Association*, **278**, 823–832.

Rogers A, Pilgrim D & Latham M (1996) **Understanding and promoting mental health: a study of familial views**. London: Health Education Authority.

Simons-Morton B G, Crump A D, Haynie D L, *et al* (1999) **Student–school bonding and adolescent problem behaviour**. *Health Education Research*, **14**, 99–107.

Tuiford S, Delaney F & Vogels M (1997) **Effectiveness of mental health promotion interventions: a review**. London: Health Education Authority.

Wight D, Abraham C & Scott S (1998) **Towards a psychosocial theoretical framework for sexual health promotion**. *Health Education Research*, **13**, 317–330.

● NEEDS ASSESSMENT ●

Barry M M, Doherty A, Hope A, *et al* (2000) **A community needs assessment for rural mental health promotion**. *Health Education Research*, **15**, 293–304.

Secker J, Armstrong C & Hill M (1999) **Young people's understanding of mental illness**. *Health Education Research*, **14**, 729–739.

● BOOKS ●

Andrews G & Henderson S (ed.) (2000) *Unmet Need in Psychiatry*. Cambridge: Cambridge University Press.

Glantz M D, Johnson J L, *et al* (eds) (1999) *Resilience and Development: Positive Life Adaptations*. New York: Kluwer Academic/Plenum Publishers.

Guimon J, Fischer W & Sartorius N (eds) (1999) *The Image of Madness: The Public Facing Mental Illness and Psychiatric Treatment*. Basel: Karger.

REFERENCES

● **STANDARDS FOR SERVICE DEVELOPMENT** ●

Association of Directors of Social Services and Royal College of Psychiatrists (1995) *Joint Statement on an Integrated Mental Health Service for Children and Adolescents*. London: Royal College of Psychiatrists.

Berger M, Hill P, Sein E, *et al* (1993) *A Proposed Core Data Set for Child and Adolescent Psychology and Psychiatry Services*. London: Association for Child Psychology and Psychiatry.

Finch J & Hill P (2000) *Health Advisory Service: Standards for Child and Adolescent Mental Health Services*. Brighton: Pavilion Publishing.

Health Quality Service in association with the King's Fund & National Children's Bureau (2000) *Standards Framework for Child and Adolescent Mental Health Services*. London: Health Quality Service.

National In-patient Child and Adolescent Psychiatry Study Research Team (2001) *Standards developed for the National In-patient Child and Adolescent Psychiatry Study*. London: The Royal College of Psychiatrists' Research Unit. (These standards form part of the Appendices to the National In-Patient Psychiatry Study submitted to the Department of Health in 2001.)

Royal College of Psychiatrists (1999) *Guidance on Staffing of Child and Adolescent In-Patient Psychiatry Units*. CR76. London: Royal College of Psychiatrists.

● **SERVICE DEVELOPMENT** ●

Berger M, Hill P, Sein E, *et al* (1993) *A Proposed Core Data Set for Child and Adolescent Psychology and Psychiatry Services*. London: Association for Child Psychology and Psychiatry.

Royal College of Psychiatrists (1999) *Guidance on Staffing of Child and Adolescent In-Patient Psychiatry Units*. CR76. London:Royal College of Psychiatrists.

● **COMMISSIONING AND FUNDING OF SERVICES** ●

Department of Health (1998) *Modernising Health and Social Services: National Priorities Guidance, 1999/00–2001/02*. Health Service Circular HSC (98)159; Local Authority Circular LAC (98)22. London: Department of Health.

—— (1999) *NHS Modernisation Fund and Mental Health Grants for Child and Adolescent Mental Health Services 1999/2000*. Health Service Circular HSC 1999/126; Local Authority Circular LAC (99)22. London: Department of Health.

——, Home Office, DfEE & National Assembly for Wales Working Together to Safeguard Children (1991) *A Guide to Interagency Working to Safeguard and Promote the Welfare of Children – Consultation Draft*. London: Department of Health.

Kurtz Z (1996) *Treating Children Well: A Guide to Using the Evidence Base in Commissioning and Managing Services for the Mental Health of Children and Young People*. London: The Mental Health Foundation.

NHS Executive (1998) *Information for Health: An Information Strategy for the Modern NHS 1998–2005: A National Strategy for Local Implementation*. London: Department of Health.

NHS Health Advisory Service (1995) *Together We Stand: Thematic Review on the Commissioning, Role and Management of Child and Adolescent Mental Health Services*. London: HMSO.

● LEGAL ASPECTS OF CAMHS ●

Department of Health (1999) *Convention on the Rights of the Child: Second Report to the UN Committee on the Rights of the Child by the United Kingdom*. London: HMSO.

House of Commons Select Health Committee (1997) *Inquiry into Mental Health Services*. London: HMSO.

● CHILDREN IN CARE AND SOCIAL SERVICES ●

Bullock R, Gooch D & Little M (1999) *Children Going Home: the Reunification of Families*. Aldershot: Ashgate Publishing.

Department of Health (1998) *Children Looked After by Local Authorities: Government Response to the Second Report of the Health Committee on Children Looked After by Local Authorities: Session 1997–98*. London: HMSO.

—— (1998) *Someone Else's Children: Inspection of Planning and Decision Making for Children Looked After and The Safety of Children Looked After*. London: Department of Health.

—— (1999) *The Government's Objectives for Children's Social Services*. London: Department of Health.

House of Commons Health Committee (1998) *Children Looked After by Local Authorities: Session 1997–98*. Health Committee Second Report: Vol. 1. London: HMSO.

Social Services Inspectorate (1993–1996) *Standards Used by the Social Services Inspectorate: Children's Services*, Vol. 2. London: Department of Health.

—— (1993–1996) *Standards Used by the Social Services Inspectorate: Children's Residential Care, Secure Accommodation and Juvenile Justice*. Vol. 3. London: Department of Health.

Utting W (1997) *People Like Us: The Report of the Review of the Safeguards for Children Living away from Home*. London: The Department of Health.

● NATIONAL REPORTS/AUDITS OF CAMHS SERVICES ●

Audit Commission (1999) *Children in Mind: Child and Adolescent Mental Health Services*. London: Audit Commission.

Kurtz Z, Thornes R & Wolkind S (1996) *Services for the Mental Health of Children and Young People in England: a National Review.* Report to the Department of Health. London: South West Thames Regional Health Authority.

—, — & — (1996) *Services for the Mental Health of Children and Young People in England: Assessment of Needs and Unmet Need*. Report to the Department of Health. London: South West Thames Regional Health Authority.

NHS Executive (1996) *NHS Psychotherapy Services in England*. London: Department of Health.

● EDUCATION ●

Department of Health and Department for Education (1995) *A Handbook on Child and Adolescent Mental Health*. Manchester: HMSO.

NACRO (1998) *Children, Schools and Crime: A Report by NACRO's Committee on Children and Crime (1996)*. London: NACRO.

OFSTED (1999) *Principles into Practice: Effective Education for Pupils with Emotional and Behavioural Difficulties (1999)*. London: HMSO.

Social Exclusion Unit, Home Office, Department of Health & Department for Education and Employment (1999) *School Inclusion: Pupil Support: The Secretary of State's Guidance on Pupil Attendance, Behaviour, Exclusion and Re-integration*. Circular No. 10/99 and 11/99. London: Department of Health.

● OTHER REPORTS ●

Chesson R & Chisholm D (eds) (1996) *Child Psychiatric Units at the Crossroads*. London: Jessica Kingsley.

Department for Education and Employment (1999) *Learning to Succeed: A New Framework for Post-16 Learning*. London: HMSO.

— (1999) *Sure Start: A Guide for Trailblazers*. London:HMSO.

Department of Health (1996) *The Patient's Charter: Services for Children and Young People*. London: HMSO.

— (1998) *Families in Focus: Evaluation of the Department of Health's Refocusing Children's Services Initiative*. London: Department of Health.

— (1999) *Consultation Draft Framework for the Assessment of Children in Need and their Families*. London: Department of Health.

Green J & Jacobs B (eds) (1998) *Inpatient Child Psychiatry*. London: Routledge.

Harrington R C, Kerfoot M, Veroluyn C, *et al* (1999) *Developing Needs-Led Child and Adult Mental Health Services: Issues and Prospects*. European Child Adolescent Psychiatry, **8**, 1–10.

Kurtz Z (ed.) (1992) *With Health in Mind: Mental Health Care for Children and Young People* (Quality Review Series). London: Action for Sick Children.

Little M & Mount K (1999) *Prevention and Early Intervention with Children in Need*. Aldershot: Ashgate Publishing.

Mental Health Foundation (1999) *Bright Futures: Promoting Children and Young People's Mental Health.* London: The Mental Health Foundation.

Pearce J & Holmes S (1995) *Health Gain Investment Programme. Technical Review Document. People with Mental Health Problems (part four): Child and Adolescent Mental Health*. London: NHS Executive Trent and Centre for Mental Health Services Department.

● USEFUL READING ●

Target M & Fonagy P (1996) **The psychological treatment of child and adolescent psychiatric disorders**. In *What Works for Whom?* (eds A Roth & P Fonagy). London: Guilford Press.

Wallace S A, Crown J M, Cox A D, *et al* (1997) *Epidemiologically Based Needs Assessment: Child and Adolescent Mental Health. Health Care Needs Assessment*. Oxford: Redcliffe Medical Press.

● THE EVIDENCE BASE FOR CAMHS ●

Carr A (ed.) (2000) *What Works with Children and Adolescents? A Critical Review of Psychological Interventions with Children, Adolescents and their Families*. London: Routledge.

Kurtz Z (1996) *Treating Children Well: A Guide to Using the Evidence Base in Commissioning and Managing Services for the Mental Health of Children and Young People*. London: The Mental Health Foundation.

Target M & Fonagy P (1996) **The psychological treatment of child and adolescent psychiatric disorders**. In *What Works for Whom?* (eds A Roth & P Fonagy). London: Guildford Press.

Appendix i: search strategies

Search strategy to identify randomised controlled trials in Medline

SILVER PLATTER FORMAT (VERSION 3.10)

From: Dickersin K, Scherer R & Lefebvre C (1994) **Identifying relevant studies for systematic reviews.** *British Medical Journal,* **309**, 1286–1291.

#1   (Subject search strategy)

#2   (TG=ANIMAL) not ((TG=HUMAN) and (TG=ANIMAL))
#3   #1 not #2

#4   RANDOMISED–CONTROLLED–TRIAL in PT
#5   CONTROLLED–CLINICAL–TRIAL in PT
#6   RANDOMISED–CONTROLLED–TRIALS
#7   RANDOM–ALLOCATION
#8   DOUBLE–BLIND–METHOD
#9   SINGLE–BLIND–METHOD

#10   CLINICAL–TRIAL in PT
#11   explode CLINICAL–TRIALS/ ALL SUBHEADINGS
#12   (clin* near trial*) in TI
#13   (clin* near trial*) in AB
#14   (singl* or doubl* or trebl* or tripl*) near (blind* or mask*)
#15   (#14 in TI) or (#14 in AB)
#16   PLACEBOS
#17   placebo* in TI
#18   placebo* in AB
#19   random* in TI
#20   random* in AB
#21   RESEARCH–DESIGN

#22   TG=COMPARATIVE–STUDY
#23   explode EVALUATION–STUDIES/ ALL SUBHEADINGS
#24   FOLLOW-UP–STUDIES
#25   PROSPECTIVE–STUDIES
#26   control* or prospectiv* or volunteer*
#27   (#26 in TI) or (#26 in AB)

#28   #4 or #5 or #6 or #7 or #8 or #9
#29   #10 or #11 or #12 or #13 or #15 or #16 or #17 or #18 or #19 or #20 or #21
#30   #22 or #23 or #24 or #25 or #27

#31   #28 or #29 or #30

#32   #3 and #31

- ○ Upper case denotes controlled vocabulary.

- ○ Lower case denotes free-text terms.

- ○ Readers wishing to run this search strategy are recommended to seek the advice of a trained medical librarian.

From: Dickersin K, Scherer R & Lefebvre C (1994) **Identifying relevant studies for systematic reviews.** *British Medical Journal,* **309**, 1286–1291.

#1   RANDOMISED CONTROLLED TRIAL.pt.
#2   CONTROLLED CLINICAL TRIAL.pt.
#3   RANDOMISED CONTROLLED TRIALS.sh.
#4   RANDOM ALLOCATION.sh.
#5   DOUBLE BLIND METHOD.sh.
#6   SINGLE–BLIND METHOD.sh.
#7   or/#1–6
#8   ANIMAL.sh. not HUMAN.sh.
#9   #7 not #8

#10   CLINICAL TRIAL.pt.
#11   exp CLINICAL TRIALS
#12   (clin$ adj25 trial$).ti,ab.
#13   ((singl$ or doubl$ or trebl$ or tripl$) adj25 (blind$ or mask$)).ti,ab.
#14   PLACEBOS.sh.
#15   placebo$.ti,ab.
#16   random$.ti,ab.
#17   RESEARCH DESIGN.sh.
#18   or/#10–17
#19   #18 not #8
#20   #19 not #9

#21   COMPARATIVE STUDY.sh.
#22   exp EVALUATION STUDIES
#23   FOLLOW UP STUDIES.sh.
#24   PROSPECTIVE STUDIES.sh.
#25   (control$ or prospectiv$ or volunteer$).ti,ab.
#26   or/#21–25
#27   #26 not #8
#28   #26 not (#9 or #20)
#29   #9 or #20 or #28

○ Upper case denotes controlled vocabulary.

○ Lower case denotes free-text terms.

○ Readers wishing to run this search strategy are recommended to seek the advice of a trained medical librarian.

OVID VERSION

● SEARCH STRATEGY 1: HIGH SENSITIVITY, LOW PRECISION ●

Best for the researcher keen to retrieve all systematic reviews while retaining a reasonable level of precision.

#1   meta.ab
#2   synthesis.ab
#3   literature.ab
#4   randomized.hw
#5   published.ab
#6   meta-analysis.pt
#7   extraction.ab
#8   trials.hw
#9   controlled.hw
#10   medline.ab
#11   selection.ab
#12   sources.ab
#13   trials.ab
#14   review.ab
#15   review.pt
#16   articles.ab
#17   reviewed.ab
#18   english.ab
#19   language.ab
#20   comment.pt
#21   letter.pt
#22   editorial.pt
#23   animal/
#24   human/
#25   #23 not (#23 and #24)
#26   (Your subject terms)
#27   #26 not (#20 or #21 or #22 or #25)
#28   or/#1–19
#29   #27 and #28

● SEARCH STRATEGY 2: HIGH PRECISION, LOW SENSITIVITY ●

Best for the busy searcher who has access only to Medline.

#1   medline.ab
#2   comment.pt
#3   letter.pt
#4   editorial.pt
#5   animal/
#6   human/
#7   #5 not (#5 and #6)
#8   (Your subject terms)
#9   #8 not (#2 or #3 or #4 or #7)
#10   #1 and #9

Adapted from Boynton J, Glanville J, McDaid D, *et al* (1998) **Identifying systematic reviews in medline: Developing an approach to search strategy design**. *Journal of Information Science*, **24**, 137–157.

#1   (Subject search strategy)
#2   (TG=ANIMAL) not ((TG=HUMAN) and (TG=ANIMAL))
#3   #1 not #2
#4   REVIEW-ACADEMIC in PT
#5   REVIEW-TUTORIAL in PT
#6   META-ANALYSIS in PT
#7   META-ANALYSIS
#8   SYSTEMATIC* near REVIEW*
#9   SYSTEMATIC* near OVERVIEW*
#10 META-ANALY* or METAANALY* or (META ANALY*)
#11 #10 in TI
#12 #10 in AB
#13 #4 or #5 or #6 or #7 or #8 or #9 or #11 or #12
#14 #3 and #13

● SEARCH STRATEGY FOR THE SENSITIVITY MAXIMISER ●

#1   (Subject search strategy)
#2   (TG=ANIMAL) not ((TG=HUMAN) and (TG=ANIMAL))
#3   #1 not #2
#4   meta in AB
#5   medline in AB
#6   synthesis in AB
#7   selection in AB
#8   literature in AB
#9   sources in AB
#10 randomized in MESH
#11 trials in AB
#12 published in AB
#13 review in AB
#14 meta-analysis in PT
#15 review in PT
#16 extraction in AB
#17 articles in AB
#18 trials in MESH
#19 reviewed in AB
#20 controlled in MESH
#21 english in AB
#22 search in AB
#23 language in AB

#24 #4 or #5 or #6 or #7 or #8 or #9 or #10 or #11 or #12 or #13 or #14 or #15 or #16 or #17 or #18 or #19 or #20 or #21 or #22 or #23
#25 #3 and #24

Appendix ii: critical appraisal tools

Critical appraisal tool: meta-analyses and systematic reviews (adapted from material produced by the Centre for Evidence-Based Mental Health)

Title of paper: ....
Author: ....
Source: ....
Date: ....

A. ARE THE RESULTS VALID?

1. Is the question clearly focused?

- What is being reviewed?
- What is the population?
- What is the exposure/intervention?
- What are the outcomes?

Comments

2. Is the search thorough? (Did the authors look for the appropriate sort of papers?)

- What bibliographic databases were used?
- What years were searched?
- What languages were searched?
- Was any hand-searching conducted or references in relevant articles obtained?
- Are the inclusion criteria appropriate – refer to study design, participants, intervention, and outcomes of interest.
- Is the inclusion process discussed?

Comments

3. **Is the validity of included studies adequately assessed?**

   ○ Reproducible, blind assessment?

   ○ Method of random selection?

   ○ Is the analysis on an intention to treat basis?

   ○ Is missing information obtained from investigators?

   ○ Is publication bias an issue?

   ○ Has methodological quality been assessed?

   Comments

B. DETAILS OF INDIVIDUAL STUDIES USED IN META-ANALYSIS OR SYSTEMATIC REVIEW

4. How many individual studies were included in the systematic review/meta-analysis?

   ○ What type of studies were included? e.g. randomised controlled trials, cohort studies, case-control studies, etc.

   ○ What are the sample sizes for each study group?

   ○ Were the patient characteristics, interventions, outcome measures and the efficacious and adverse results discussed/presented for each study? What were they?

   Comments

5. In what countries were the treatment studies conducted?

   Comments

6. If medication was used, what were the dosages of medication used for each study?

   Comments

7. What was the duration of treatment (give the range)?

Comments

8. Are the studies focused on boys or girls or both?

Comments

9. Were the children receiving concomitant medication/treatment?

Comments

C. WHAT ARE THE RESULTS?

10. How big is the overall effect?

○ On what scale is the effect measured? (odds ratio, number needed to treat?)

Comments

11. Are the results consistent from study to study?

○ How sensitive are the results to changes in the way the review was done?

Comments

12. If the results of the review have been combined, was it reasonable to do so?

○ Were the results similar from study to study?

○ Are the results of the included studies clearly displayed?

○ Are the results of the different studies similar?

○ Are the reasons for any variations in results discussed?

Comments

13. How precise are the results?

○ Does the lower confidence limit include clinically relevant effects?

○ Does the upper confidence limit exclude clinically relevant effects?

Comments

D. INTERPRETATION OF THE RESULTS – WILL THEY HELP IN MAKING DECISIONS ABOUT PATIENTS?

---

14. Do conclusions flow from evidence that is reviewed?

Comments

---

15. Are subgroup analyses interpreted cautiously?

Comments

---

16. Can the conclusions and data be generalised to other settings? (Is the number needed to treat stated or should it be calculated?)

Comments

---

17. Were all important outcomes considered?

Comments

---

18. Are the benefits worth the harms and the costs?

Comments

ADDITIONAL COMMENTS

Title of paper:
Author:
Source:
Date:

A. ARE THE RESULTS OF THIS TRIAL VALID?

1. **Are you using the right research paper to answer your particular question?**

   Comments

2. **Was the group of patients clearly defined?**

   Consider:

   - the population studied (age, gender, setting, country)

   - comorbidity (note if any children were excluded from the study)

   - classification used

   - outcomes measured.

   Comments

3. **Was the assignment of patients to treatments randomised?**

   - Was the randomisation list concealed?

   Comments

4. **Were all patients who entered the trial accounted for at its conclusion?**

   Comments

5. **Were they analysed in the groups to which they were randomised?**

   Comments

6. Were patients and clinicians kept 'blind' to which treatment was being received?

Comments

7. Aside from the experimental treatment, were the groups treated equally?

Comments

8. If a cross-over design was used, were attempts made to reduce the carry-over effects?

○ Did the authors acknowledge that this was a potential problem?

○ Was an appropriate wash-out period used?

Comments

B. WHAT ARE THE RESULTS?

9. How large was the treatment effect?

○ See Guidance: calculating number needed to treat (page 193)

Comments

10. How precise is the estimate of treatment effect?

○ See Guidance: calculating confidence intervals (page 195)

Comments

C. WHAT ARE THE IMPLICATIONS OF THIS PAPER FOR LOCAL PRACTICE?

11. Are the results of this study generalisable to your patients?

○ Does your patient resemble those in the study?

○ What are your patient's preferences?

○ Are there alternative treatments available?

Comments

'Number needed to treat' (NNT) represents the number of patients you need to treat in order to prevent one negative outcome.

A worked example is included on the following page.

2.1 ESTABLISH THE CONTROL EVENT RATE

The control event rate (CER) is the proportion of patients in the study's control group experiencing the observed negative event.

Enter the CER for your study in the box:

CER =

2.2 ESTABLISH THE EXPERIMENTAL EVENT RATE

The experimental event rate (EER) is the proportion of patients in the study's experimental group (i.e. the group receiving the experimental treatment) experiencing the observed negative event.

Enter the EER for your study in the box:

EER =

2.3 CALCULATE THE ABSOLUTE RISK REDUCTION

The absolute risk reduction (ARR) is the absolute difference in the risk of an adverse outcome between the control group and the experimental group. It is calculated by deducting the EER from the CER.

Perform this calculation now:

ARR =   **(CER from above) –**   **(EER from above) =**

2.4 CALCULATE THE NUMBER NEEDED TO TREAT

The NNT is calculated by dividing the ARR into 1 and multiplying the result by 100. Perform this calculation now:

NNT = 1 /   **(ARR from above) x 100 =**

NNTs: worked example

SAMPLE DATA

A population of 200 patients was divided into an experimental and a control group with 100 patients in each. The experimental group was given haloperidol in order to prevent recurrence of psychotic episodes. Ten patients in the experimental group experienced a psychotic episode during the period of the trial. Thirty-five patients in the control group experienced a psychotic episode during the period of the trial.

1. ESTABLISH THE CER

35 patients experienced the event out of a population of 100, therefore the CER will be 35%.

CER = 35%

2. ESTABLISH THE EER?

10 patients experienced the event out of a population of 100, therefore the EER will be 10%.

EER = 10%

3. CALCULATE THE ARR

In this example, the CER equals 35% and the EER equals 10%.

ARR = 35 (CER from above) – 10 (EER from above) = 25%

4. CALCULATE THE NNT

In our sample data, the ARR equals 25%.

NNT = 1/25 (ARR from above) x 100 = 4

The confidence interval (CI) gives the range within which we would expect the true value of a statistical measure to lie.

Most research studies use a CI of 95%; for example, an NNT of 10 with a 95% CI of 5 to 15 would give us 95% confidence that the true NNT value was between 5 and 15.

3.1 THE FORMULA

The formula for calculating a 95% Confidence Interval on an NNT is:

$$\pm 1.96 \sqrt{\frac{\text{CER} \times (1 - \text{CER})}{n \text{ of contol patients}} + \frac{\text{EER} \times (1 - \text{EER})}{n \text{ of experimental patients}}}$$

Please note: in the formula the CER and EER are expressed as fractions, rather than percentages. For example, a 25% CER is expressed as 0.25.

$$\pm 1.96 \sqrt{\frac{\ldots \times (1 - \ldots)}{\ldots} + \frac{\ldots \times (1 - \ldots)}{\ldots}} = \ldots$$

This will give you the percentage range within which the truly accurate NNT can be found. The smaller the percentage, the more confident you can be that the NNT is accurate.

Title of paper: . . . .

Author: . . . .

Source: . . . .

Date: . . . .

A. ARE THE RECOMMENDATIONS IN THIS GUIDELINE VALID?

1. Were all important decision options and outcomes clearly specified?

2. Was the evidence relevant to each decision option identified, validated and combined in a sensible and explicit way?

3. Are the relative preferences that key stakeholders attach to the outcomes of decisions (including benefits, risks and costs) identified and explicitly considered?

4. Is the guideline resistant to clinically sensible variations in practice?

Comments

B. IS THIS GUIDELINE POTENTIALLY USEFUL?

5. Does this guideline offer an opportunity for significant improvement in the quality of health care practice?

○ Is there a large variation in current practice?

○ Does the guideline contain new evidence (or old evidence not yet acted upon) that could have an important impact on management?

○ Would the guideline affect the management of so many people, or concern individuals at such high risk, or involve such high costs that even small changes in practice could have major impacts on health outcomes or resources?

Comments

6. **What barriers exist to its implementation?**

   ○ Can they be overcome?

7. **Can you collaborate with key colleagues to implement the guideline?**

8. **Can you meet the variety of conditions that will determine the success or failure of implementing the guideline? For example:**

   ○ Has the evidence been collated by a respected body (e.g. a rigorously developed clinical practice guideline from a Royal College)?

   ○ Are local opinion leaders already implementing the strategy?

   ○ Have you received consistent information from all relevant sources?

   ○ Has there been an opportunity for individual discussions about the strategy with a respected colleague/authority?

   ○ Has a 'user-friendly' format for the guidelines been developed? (It may require local adaptation.)

   ○ Can you implement the guideline within a target group of clinicians (without the need for extensive outside collaboration)?

   ○ Does the guideline represent a conflict of interest with patient and community expectations, economic incentives, administrative incentives, etc.?

Comments

ADDITIONAL COMMENTS

Criteria for the evaluation of qualitative research papers (adapted from the British Sociological Association Medical Sociology Group Guidelines, 1996)

1. Are the methods of the research appropriate to the nature of the question being asked?

Comments

○ Does the research seek to understand processes or structures, or illuminate subjective experiences or meanings?

○ Are the categories or groups being examined of a type that cannot be pre-selected, or the possible outcomes cannot be specified in advance?

○ Could a quantitative approach have addressed the issue better?

2. Is the connection to an existing body of knowledge or theory clear?

Comments

○ Is there adequate reference to the literature?

○ Does the work cohere with, or critically address, existing theory?

METHODS

3. Are there clear accounts of the criteria used for the selection of subjects for study, and of the data collection and analysis?

Comments

4. Is the selection of cases or participants theoretically justified?

○ The unit of research may be people, or events, institutions, samples of natural behaviour, conversations, written material, etc. In any case, while random sampling may not be appropriate, is it nevertheless clear what population the sample refers to?

○ Is consideration given to whether the units chosen were unusual in some important way?

5. Does the sensitivity of the methods match the needs of the research questions?

- ○ Does the method accept the implications of an approach that respects the perceptions of those studied?

- ○ To what extent are any definitions or agendas taken for granted, rather than being critically examined or left open?

- ○ Are the limitations of any structured interview method considered?

6. Has the relationship between field-workers and subjects been considered, and is there evidence that the research was presented and explained to its subjects?

- ○ If more than one worker was involved, has comparability been considered?

- ○ Is there evidence about how the subjects perceived the research?

- ○ Is there evidence about how any group processes were conducted?

7. Was the data collection and record-keeping systematic?

- ○ Were careful records kept?

- ○ Is the evidence available for independent examination?

- ○ Were full records or transcripts of conversations used if appropriate?

Comments

8. **Is reference made to accepted procedures for analysis?**

    ○ Is it clear how the analysis was done? (Detailed repetition of how to perform standard procedures ought not to be expected.)

    ○ Has its reliability been considered, ideally by independent repetition?

9. **How systematic is the analysis?**

    ○ What steps were taken to guard against selectivity in the use of data?

    ○ In research with individuals, is it clear that there has not been selection of some cases and ignoring of less interesting ones? In group research, are all categories of opinion taken into account?

10. **Is there adequate discussion of how themes, concepts and categories were derived from the data?**

    ○ It is sometimes inevitable that externally given or predetermined descriptive categories are used, but have they been examined for their real meaning or any possible ambiguities?

11. **Is there adequate discussion of the evidence both for and against the researcher's arguments?**

    ○ Are negative data given?

    ○ Has there been any search for cases that might refute the conclusions?

12. **Have measures been taken to test the validity of the findings?**

    ○ Have methods such as feeding them back to the respondents, triangulation, or procedures such as grounded theory been used?

Comments

13. Have any steps been taken to see whether the analysis would be comprehensible to the participants, if this is possible and relevant?

- ○ Has the meaning of their accounts been explored with respondents?

- ○ Have apparent anomalies and contradictions been discussed with them, rather than assumptions been made?

Comments

PRESENTATION

14. Is the research clearly contextualised?

- ○ Has all the relevant information about the setting and subjects been supplied?

- ○ Are the variables being studied integrated in their social context, rather then abstracted and decontextualised?

15. Are the data presented systematically?

- ○ Are quotations, fieldnotes, etc. identified in a way that enables the reader to judge the range of evidence used?

16. Is a clear distinction made between the data and their interpretation?

- ○ Do the conclusions follow from the data?

17. Is sufficient of the original evidence presented to satisfy the reader of the relationship between the evidence and the conclusions?

- ○ Although the presentation of discursive data is always going to require more space than numerical data, is the paper as concise as possible?

Comments

18. Is the author's own position clearly stated?

○ Is the researcher's perspective described?

○ Has the researcher examined his or her own role, possible bias and influence on the research?

19. Are the results credible and appropriate?

○ Do they address the research question(s)?

○ Are they plausible and coherent?

○ Are they important, either theoretically or practically, or trivial?

Comments

ETHICS

20. Have ethical issues been adequately considered?

○ Has the issue of confidentiality been adequately dealt with?

○ Have the consequences of the research – including establishing relationships with the subjects, raising expectations, changing behaviour, etc. – been considered?

Comments

REFERENCE

British Sociological Association Medical Sociology Group (1996) *British Sociological Association Medical Sociology Group Guidelines. Criteria for Evaluation of Qualitative Research Papers*. London: Medical Sociology Group of the British Sociological Association.

Appendix iii: fax back to FOCUS

We hope the papers that we have included in this book will be of value to people who are keen to learn more about their subjects of interest. Please help us keep this record up-to-date by faxing any examples of secondary research that we may have missed. Thank you.

To: FOCUS Office

Fax: 020 7227 0850

Date:

From:

Subject

Title of article

Source (please provide a full reference)

Systematic review/meta-analyses or clinical guideline or report?
(Please circle appropriate heading).

If you do not have access to a fax machine please send this form to:

The FOCUS Project
The Royal College of Psychiatrists' Research Unit
6th Floor, 83 Victoria Street
London SW1H 0HW